About the Author

Alex de Waal is a writer and activist on African issues. He is a fellow of the Global Equity Initiative, Harvard; director of the Social Science Research Council program on AIDS and social transformation; and a director of Justice Africa in London. In his twenty-year career he has studied the social, political and health dimensions of famine, war, genocide and the HIV/AIDS epidemic, especially in the Horn of Africa and the Great Lakes. He has been at the forefront of mobilizing African and international responses to these problems. His books include *Famine that Kills: Darfur Sudan* (Oxford University Press, first edition 1989, revised 2004), *Famine Crimes: Politics and the Disaster Relief Industry in Africa* (James Currey, 1997), *Islamism and Its Enemies in the Horn of Africa* (Hurst, 2004) and (with Julie Flint) *Darfur: A Short History of a Long War* (Zed Books, 2005).

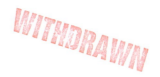

AFRICAN ARGUMENTS
A new series from Zed Books
in association with the International African Institute

African Arguments is a series of short books about Africa today. Aimed at the growing number of students and general readers who want to know more about the continent, these books intend to highlight many of the longer-term strategic as well as immediate political issues confronting the African continent. They will get to the heart of why Africa is the way it is and how it is changing. The books are scholarly but engaged, substantive as well as topical.

Series editors
ALEX DE WAAL, Global Equity Initiative, Harvard University
RICHARD DOWDEN, Executive Director, Royal African Society
TAJUDEEN ABDUL RAHEEM, Director, Justice Africa

Editorial board
EMMANUEL AKYEAMPONG, Professor of History, Harvard University
TIM ALLEN, London School of Economics
ALCINDA HONWANA, The Open University
ABDUL MOHAMMED, InterAfrica Group

Titles already published
Julie Flint and Alex de Waal, *Darfur: A Short History of a Long War*
Tim Allen, *Trial Justice: The International Criminal Court and the Lord's Resistance Army*
Alex de Waal, *AIDS and Power: Why there is no political crisis – yet*

In preparation
Tajudeen Abdul Raheem, *The African Union*

**African Arguments is published by Zed Books and the IAI
with the support of the following organizations:**

Global Equity Initiative The Global Equity Initiative seeks to advance the understanding and tackle the challenges of global inequitable development. Located at Harvard University, it has international collaborative research programmes on security, health, capabilities and philanthropy.
www.fas.harvard.edu/~acgei

InterAfrica Group The InterAfrica Group is the regional centre for dialogue on issues of development, democracy, conflict resolution and humanitarianism in the Horn of Africa. It was founded in 1988 and is based in Addis Ababa; it has programmes supporting democracy in Ethiopia and partnership with the African Union and IGAD.

International African Institute The International African Institute's principal aim is to promote scholarly understanding of Africa, notably its changing societies, cultures and languages. Founded in 1926 and based in London, it supports a range of seminars and publications including the journal *Africa*.
www.iaionthe.net

Justice Africa Justice Africa initiates and supports African civil society activities in support of peace, justice and democracy in Africa. Founded in 1999, it has a range of activities in support of peace in the Horn of Africa, HIV/AIDS and democracy, and the African Union.
www.justiceafrica.org

Royal African Society Now more than a hundred years old, the Royal African Society is today Britain's leading organization promoting Africa's cause. Through its journal, *African Affairs*, and by organizing meetings, discussions and other activities, the Society strengthens links between Africa and Britain and encourages understanding of Africa and its relations with the rest of the world.
www.royalafricansociety.org

Social Science Research Council The Social Science Research Council brings necessary knowledge to public issues. Founded in 1923 and based in New York, it brings together researchers, practitioners and policymakers on every continent.
www.ssrc.org

AIDS and Power

Why there is no political crisis — yet

_____

Alex de Waal

Zed Books
LONDON & NEW YORK

David Philip
CAPE TOWN

in association with the
International African Institute
and the
Royal African Society

AIDS and Power: Why there is no political crisis – yet was first published
in association with the International African Institute and
the Royal African Society in 2006 by

In Southern Africa: David Philip (an imprint of New Africa Books),
99 Garfield Road, Claremont 7700, South Africa

In the rest of the world: Zed Books Ltd, 7 Cynthia Street, London N1 9JF, UK,
and Room 400, 175 Fifth Avenue, New York, NY 10010, USA

www.zedbooks.co.uk
www.iaionthe.net
www.royalafricansociety.org

Designed and typeset in Monotype Joanna
by Long House Publishing Services, Cumbria, UK
Cover designed by Andrew Corbett
Printed and bound in Malta by Gutenberg Press Ltd

Distributed in the USA exclusively by Palgrave Macmillan, a division of
St Martin's Press, LLC, 175 Fifth Avenue, New York, NY 10010

A catalogue record for this book is available from the British Library
Library of Congress Cataloging-in-Publication Data available

ISBN 1 84277 706 8 Hb
ISBN 1 84277 707 6 Pb
ISBN 978 1 84277 706 0 Hb
ISBN 978 1 84277 707 7 Pb

Contents

Acknowledgements

Many people have contributed to this book. Preparatory research was done by Jacob Bor, Ephraim Kimoto, Kintu Nyago, Roxanne Rawson, Charles Wendo and Samantha Willan through a Justice Africa research programme supported by the Cultural Cooperation, Education and Research Department of the Netherlands Ministry of Foreign Affairs. This book draws heavily on work done within the African civil society Governance and AIDS Initiative (GAIN), especially by Ngonzi Kiiza, Jacinta Maingi and Alastair Roderick, supported by the Open Society Foundation of South Africa. The analysis of Uganda owes much to Tim Allen and Joseph Tumushabe. Parts of the analysis in Chapter 4 were presented at a conference at the Clingendael Institute in the Hague in May 2005, and benefited from the discussion, especially points made by Laetitia van den Assum, Tsadkan Gebre Tensae and Bill Brady. Useful critiques and comments on the text have come from Dennis Altman, Tony Barnett, Richard Dowden, Jennifer Klot, Bob Mattes, Robert Molteno, Per Strand and Alan Whiteside. Initial research for this book was made possible by grants to Justice Africa from ICCO (Netherlands) and KIOS (Finland), which also provided a grant for copies to be distributed in Africa.

1

A Manageable Catastrophe

Perhaps the most extraordinary aspect of the African AIDS epidemic is its limited social and political effect. This is a disease which in a number of countries will be the cause of death of half the population.... It has increased the mortality levels of adults in their prime, 20–40 years, to pre-modern levels. At any one time one third of the people one meets in cities like Harare or Blantyre are infected and have at the most only a few years to live.... The additional death rate because of the epidemic, up to ten per thousand annually in some countries, is of a similar magnitude to the experience of France during the First World War, an experience that traumatized the French. Yet East and Southern Africa are not traumatized. Governments are not threatened by accusations of mishandling the epidemic. Not a single protest demonstration has occurred. Life goes on in a surprisingly normal way. There has not even been any very marked change in sexual behaviour, and society is not dominated by government demands that there should be. There is no paranoia and little in the way of new religious or death cults. In some ways it is very impressive.

John Caldwell, 1997[1]

Recently a peaceful demonstration in [Queenstown, South Africa] by AIDS patients begging for drugs to treat their otherwise fatal disease was broken up by riot police. The demonstrators, most of whom were HIV-positive women, were beaten, and 10 were shot. The next day in Moscow, people infected with HIV chained themselves to government buildings, also demanding access to life-sparing medicines. We are entering a new stage in the world's great modern plague in which long-complacent governments are awakening to discover that the HIV virus, first noticed in 1981, now threatens to foment social unrest, undermine state authority, weaken armies, challenge economies and reverse hundreds of billions of dollars' worth of development investment.

Laurie Garrett, 2005[2]

At present levels of infection, about one sixth of all the people in sub-Saharan Africa will contract HIV in their lifetimes. But the epidemic does not threaten the continent's rulers – democratic or otherwise. AIDS kills millions every year, more than war and famine combined. It kills adults, devastating families and leaving orphans. But governments are not being overthrown. Indeed, with a few exceptions such as Botswana, African leaders' responses lack urgency and scale. Governments find resources for many things, but AIDS programmes are rarely near the top of their list. There are straightforward reasons for this neglect. African electors are not demanding that their governments make AIDS a priority. Society is neither collapsing nor being transformed in revolutionary ways. African rulers, with a sound appreciation of how power functions, know that they won't be removed from office or even face political threats on account of AIDS. John Caldwell is right.

Laurie Garrett says that 'this is the Black Death'.[3] By invoking this spectre and predicting social meltdown in Africa, she wants to frighten powerful governments into massive and urgent action. This drumbeat of doomsaying has made an impact in

Washington DC and New York, but not in Africa, where pundits' forecasts of collapse are routinely discounted and fear of an abstract apocalypse has long since failed to spur political action.

This book argues that African governments, civil society organizations and international institutions have proved remarkably effective at managing the HIV/AIDS epidemic in a way that minimizes political threats. In doing so, they have adopted a model of response to AIDS that focuses on process rather than outcome – chiefly the smooth and coordinated functioning of their own institutions, but also adherence to certain principles, some of which are based on evidence, and some on faith. These process indicators, such as UNAIDS's 'three ones',[4] are rigorously assessed. Encouragingly for democrats, this process emphasizes human rights and the participation of civil society leaders, and it has thereby ensured that democracy in African is not threatened by the epidemic and may even be strengthened. With a few important exceptions where different intersecting stresses come together, AIDS is unlikely to cause socio-political crisis.

Providing antiretroviral treatment to people living with HIV and AIDS is the most effective means of managing AIDS. It is an easily measured service-delivery operation. It is a humanitarian activity that prolongs people's lives and reduces the social and economic impacts of the disease. Treatment has a ready constituency – people living with HIV and AIDS – and it is unsurprising that it has recently received a great deal of political energy and commitment. Amid the current enthusiasm for scaling up treatment, it is easy to overlook the fact that it will not roll back the epidemic.

The HIV/AIDS epidemic is being managed, not solved. For HIV/AIDS to be rolled back, the right political incentives for HIV prevention need to be in place. The first requirement is a good and rapid measure of success. Astonishingly, the only good indicator – *incidence* of HIV infections – simply isn't measured. Instead, HIV *prevalence* – the total number of existing infections –

Table 1.1: Life expectancy, related measures and HIV prevalence for selected countries

Country	Additional life expectancy at 20 years e20	Life expectancy at birth e0	Adult HIV rate 2002 (%)	Under 5 mortality per 1,000 5q0
Japan	61.9	81.7	<0.1	4
United States	57.9	77.4	0.6	8
Brazil	52.4	68.7	0.7	35
Bangladesh	48.6	62.4	0.2	69
Chad	41.1	48.3	4.8	200
Niger	39.6	46.4	1.2	262
South Africa	**35.5**	**45.7**	**21.5**	**66**
Sierra Leone	33.0	37.4	7.0	283
Malawi	**30.7**	**37.5**	**14.2**	**178**
Zambia	**27.3**	**36.5**	**16.5**	**182**
Botswana	**24.9**	**38.0**	**37.3**	**112**

Sources: Col. 1: WHO Statistical Information System, *Life Tables for 191 Countries*; Cols 2, 4, 5: WHO, *World Health Report*, 2005; Col. 3: UNAIDS, *Report on the Global AIDS Epidemic*, 2004; Col. 6: Population Division of the Dept. of Economic and Social Affairs of the UN, 2004; UNAIDS, 2004; Cols 7–8: Population Division, 2004.

is monitored rather inadequately. Prevalence can go up and down for many reasons, including changes in surveillance methods, population migration and deaths of people living with AIDS, as well as new infections. Relying on prevalence figures, we have only the vaguest grasp of whether prevention measures are having any impact at all. Even if African publics and international activists wanted to call governments and agencies to account for their performance, they do not have the tools to do so. A government's political commitment to preventing HIV/AIDS consists solely in a promise to implement a package of internationally recommended prevention strategies. There is no discernible system of political rewards for success and penalties for failure, so we should not be surprised that governments and international institutions have not made much progress in preventing HIV infections.

% of total deaths under 5 years	% of total deaths attributed to AIDS	Adult deaths per 1,000 45q15 (women)	Adult deaths per 1,000 45q15 (men)	
<0.1	<0.1	45	96	
1.0	0.6	82	139	
11	1.3	129	240	
24	<0.1	258	251	
48	9.9	444	513	
68	1.8	477	508	
10	**49.1**	**579**	**642**	
56	10.0	517	597	
36	**31.6**	**615**	**652**	
33	**34.9**	**685**	**719**	
12	**75.0**	**839**	**850**	

Life Expectancy and Public Opinion

Caldwell's sketch of AIDS's demographics remains broadly correct today. Table 1.1 ranks selected countries on the basis of the additional life expectancy of a 20-year-old. Countries with HIV prevalence over 10 per cent of adults are marked in bold.

Column 1 shows that a young adult in the United States in 2006 can expect to live until nearly eighty; a Zambian teenager to less than fifty (e20 is the number of additional years a 20-year-old can expect to live, while e0 is life expectancy at birth). From a class of 100 ninth-grade American girls aged fifteen, 90 will see their sixtieth birthdays. Less than one third of their counterparts in Malawi can expect to live that long (45q15 is the probability of a fifteen-year-old dying in the next 45 years of

life). A Batswana teenager today has a lifetime chance of contracting HIV of well over 75 per cent.[5] Today's generation faces a
greater inequity in global life chances than its predecessors, and
this is increasingly due to adult mortality and not child deaths
(column 4 shows child mortality: 5q0 is the number of children
who die before they reach five). Young adults in developed
countries expect to live longer and more prosperous lives than
their parents. In much of sub-Saharan Africa, the opposite is true,
and this reversal is very recent. Just fifteen years ago, Zambians
could expect to live to almost 60, and life expectancies in poor
countries were closing the gap on the wealthy AIDS-impacted
countries are losing ground fast. Between 2000 and 2004, South
Africans' life expectancy fell behind that of people in Chad and
Niger.

There have been wobbles on the path to development before.
This is different. Africa's shocking life expectancy regression is
due overwhelmingly to AIDS. A famine lasts a couple of years and
leaves its scars, but even the worst – such as China's 'Great Leap
Forward' disaster of 1958–61, which killed perhaps 30 million
people – are demographically absorbed within a decade or so.
AIDS is here to stay: we must speak of an 'AIDS endemic'. We just
don't know if HIV infections will 'stabilize' at a particular
prevalence level, and what that level might be. We don't know if
levels will fluctuate, with future 'waves' of infection – perhaps
driven by new viral strains – rolling through the population. 'We
are threatened with extinction,' Botswana's President Mogae told
the UN General Assembly in 2001. 'People are dying in chillingly
high numbers. It is a crisis of the first magnitude.'[6] Strictly
speaking, Mogae is wrong: demographic modelling suggests that
even very high prevalence levels – up to 40 per cent or so – can
be sustained indefinitely without a fall in the absolute numbers
of a population. At that prevalence, the great majority of adults
will end their lives early to AIDS. Today's crash in life expectancy
will not be quickly reversed. But Mogae poses a question of vast

importance: how can social order be sustained under such protracted calamity?

But across eastern and southern Africa, AIDS does not head the population's list of priorities. The Afrobarometer public opinion surveys show that AIDS is a concern to African publics but that it rarely ranks at or near the top.[7] The finding is consistent. Begun in 1999 by the University of Cape Town, the Afrobarometer is the first systematic attempt to poll public opinion in the continent. Three rounds of general surveys, including questions on a wide range of public issues, have been conducted in a growing number of countries. The first survey covered 12 countries in eastern and southern Africa. The 2004 round covered 18 countries, ranging as far as Senegal and Madagascar. The surveys include questions on attitudes to AIDS, personal experience with AIDS, and – significantly for this inquiry – how people regard government policy. It is an extraordinarily rich dataset.

To anyone familiar with the figures for HIV prevalence in southern and eastern Africa and some of the scenarios for crisis these imply, what is most striking about the Afrobarometer data is how low concern about AIDS ranks. In the 1999 survey few people named HIV/AIDS as a priority for the government's agenda.[8] Instead they ranked government action on unemployment, poverty, crime, education and general health improvements as higher priorities. In the second round (2002), the rankings were similar. South Africans put unemployment at the head of 'the most important problems facing the country that the government ought to address'. Despite growing concern, AIDS ranked lower.

Location matters: Afrobarometer data show diverging profiles of public opinion on AIDS in different countries. For example, South Africans are much more critical of their government's performance than Batswana. Unlike the monolithic pandemic portrayed in the aggregate figures, each society sees HIV/AIDS in its own way. Everywhere, there is concern over AIDS, but it is

Table 1.2: Priorities for African publics*

Botswana		Uganda		Malawi		Mozambique		South Africa	
Unempl.	61	Poverty	45	Famine	54	Unempl.	60	Unempl.	80
Poverty	36	Health	34	Poverty	35	Health	35	Crime	33
AIDS	29	Unempl.	26	Farming	32	Education	28	Poverty	29
Education	21	Education	25	Economy	22	Poverty	25	**AIDS**	27
Farming	14	Water	17	Health	22	Famine	13	Education	14
Health	13	Farming	16	Unempl.	20	**AIDS**	13	Corruption	12
Crime	12	Economy	13	Water	16	Farming	11	Health	10
Economy	12	Crime	12	Education	16	Water	11	Famine	9
Famine	10	Corruption	11	Crime	12	Crime	10	Water	8
Water	6	Roads	9	Roads	6	Corruption	6	Economy	7
Corruption	3	**AIDS**	7	Corruption	4	Economy	6	Farming	3
Infrastruct.	3	Famine	5	**AIDS**	3	Roads	4	Roads	2

* As percentages of respondents mentioning an issue in the top three priorities.

Source: Afrobarometer, 2002 'What are the most important problems facing this country that the government should address?'

usually hidden in a thicket of other worries that shadow people's lives. This is our starting point: if African voters are not concerned with HIV/AIDS, it follows that the politicians they vote into office will not be impelled to make AIDS a priority.

Structure of This Book

The four substantive chapters of this book (chapters 2–5) address a series of issues around the politics of HIV/AIDS, relating it in turn to public concern and imagining, activism and civil society, threats to social and political functioning, and power relations.

Chapter 2 begins with the larger question posed by the Afrobarometer data, 'why a pandemic that has caused such a widespread sense of personal loss in many countries, and is imposing significant burdens on households, is not named as a priority public issue more frequently?'[9] This is framed around the issue of denial, construed first as a simple refusal to recognize reality and then (more interestingly) as the determined effort to reconstruct a 'normal' social and moral order in the midst of the epidemic. Key to overcoming denial is the role of the media – not as a purveyor of messages about AIDS but as a news source that provokes discussion.

Chapter 3 examines the nature of civil society and activist mobilization around AIDS in Africa. Beginning with a close examination of the violence at the Treatment Action Campaign (TAC) protest in Queenstown, South Africa in July 2005, this chapter illustrates how HIV/AIDS is *not* a harbinger of revolution or political crisis. For different reasons, the key stakeholders in the public representation of HIV/AIDS – including AIDS activists themselves – have not framed the issue as a challenge to the legitimacy of governments. Since its foundation in 1998, South Africa's TAC has become the continent's most influential AIDS activist organization. Facing a government with an overtly denialist position on AIDS, the TAC has nonetheless framed its objectives as fulfilling the provisions of the South African constitution, not overthrowing it. Moreover, AIDS activism has undergone its own revolution, working within global structures of governance and assistance.

Popular mobilization is not the only way in which AIDS could challenge governments. If the disease were to destroy administrative capacity, breed a generation of delinquent youth or unleash social and economic crises such as famine, it could bring down democracies. Chapter 4 examines these possibilities, and finds them improbable. The evidence for catastrophic socio-economic repercussions is as yet slender. But we must be alert to the more subtle and far-reaching ways in which AIDS can influence the trajectory of social development.

Perhaps more importantly, African rulers have found means of minimizing the dangers posed by AIDS, and indeed turning the epidemic to political advantage. A case study of this is elaborated in Chapter 5, which examines the Ugandan 'success story' through the lens of President Yoweri Museveni's political career. This chapter also turns to how the emerging international AIDS apparatus is changing the matrices of power in Africa, creating new forms of both accountability and dependency. As vast treatment programmes are rolled out, consuming a large proportion of aid to Africa, governance will change yet again. Today's norms and structures provide for good representation by civil society leaders, including AIDS activists.

But we should not mistake managing the political and social threats emanating from the AIDS epidemic for an effective response to the immense human tragedy of HIV/AIDS itself. The concluding chapter reminds us how little we know about the reasons for Uganda's decline in HIV prevalence during the 1990s and suggests that we still lack the kind of evidence we need if we are to be able to design effective policies and programmes to overcome HIV/AIDS. We are not seriously demanding that our leaders prevent HIV infections, and we should not be surprised that they are failing to do so.

2

Denial and How It Is Overcome

Private Experience and Public Concern

According to any objective calculus, HIV/AIDS is the greatest contemporary threat to African lives and livelihoods. The continent, it seems, is in a state of collective denial.

Personal denial is encountered everywhere – individuals denying that they or their partners have HIV in the face of good reason to believe that they might be infected. But very few people dispute the existence of the HIV/AIDS pandemic altogether. Across the continent, there are billboards and radio messages, statements from politicians and church leaders, news stories and NGO programmes, all hammering home the message that HIV/AIDS is a risk. In the 2003 round of the Afrobarometer survey, more than half of respondents in Kenya, Malawi, Namibia, Tanzania, Uganda and Zambia reported that they had lost at least one close friend or relative to AIDS.[1] In Uganda it was 85 per cent and the median number of friends or relatives said to have died of AIDS was five. What these figures tell us is that most people readily accept that HIV/AIDS exists, even though many refuse to accept the possibility that they might have contracted the virus.

South Africa is a special case. Here, just 18 per cent reported a personal loss. One of those who refuses to acknowledge a personal loss is President Thabo Mbeki, who has publicly said that he does not know anyone who has died of AIDS. Mbeki's position – still lacking a rational explanation – legitimizes a variety of denialist views, including the scientific or epidemiological denialism propounded by a small number of 'dissident' academics, who claim that HIV does not cause AIDS, that AIDS does not exist, or that the statistics for HIV prevalence are erroneous or fraudulent. But even with presidential endorsement, few South Africans support scientific denialism.[2]

One obvious explanation of the low level of public concern is that HIV prevalence is an abstraction. The time-lag between infection with HIV and illness with AIDS is so long – eight to ten years – that a new epidemic consists mostly of symptom-less HIV infection rather than visible sickness and death from AIDS. The epidemic started late in South Africa and the country has only recently begun to experience mounting numbers of illnesses and deaths, which could help explain the low numbers of people reporting a personal loss. Successive Afrobarometer surveys show how AIDS is climbing South Africans' ladder of concern. The number of South Africans who agreed that 'AIDS [is] the most important problem' doubled from 13 to 26 per cent over three years to 2003,[3] and more people who experienced a personal loss due to AIDS identified the disease as an important political issue.[4] Statistically, the relationship between personal loss and naming AIDS as a political issue is significant, but weak. In Namibia concern has measurably increased also.[5]

There are many individual cases in which a person has become an activist on finding out that he or she is HIV-positive, or through bereavement due to AIDS. Some instances are described in the next chapter. But this does not seem to be a general phenomenon. Even where the epidemic is two decades old and almost everyone has lost a friend or relative – as in most East

African countries – people tend not to register AIDS as a public priority. The proportion of Zambians and Malawians who cite HIV/AIDS as an issue for government action remains very low at 3–4 per cent. In Tanzania the number rose sharply from 1 to 12 per cent between 2000 and 2003 – a rise that cannot be explained by bereavements, which began rising sharply in the 1980s. The statistical relationship between personal loss and naming AIDS as a political issue is not significant in most countries. South Africa's exceptional status might reflect the way in which the Treatment Action Campaign has succeeded in mobilizing people living with HIV and AIDS. Lack of personal exposure to AIDS does not explain lack of public concern.

There is a missing link. People overwhelmingly acknowledge that there is an AIDS epidemic, but do not take the next step of accepting the consequences. This is familiar territory for those concerned with trying to change risky sexual behaviour: know-ledge about how HIV is transmitted and the dangers of certain kinds of practices does not seem to translate into behavioural change. In a parallel way, we need to understand why acknow-ledging an *epidemic* does not lead people to demand *policy change*.

In his study of how individuals and societies deny knowledge of atrocities, Stan Cohen distinguishes between three types of denial. The first is 'literal': people simply refuse to accept what is happening. This is rare. A second is 'interpretative', in which the basic outline of events is acknowledged but the patterns and meanings are disputed. The last is 'implicatory' denial, in which people absolve themselves of responsibility for what has happen-ed.[6] Cohen also develops a sequence of forms of denial, moving from outright denial to discrediting, renaming and finally justification or 'normalization'. In the higher stages of denial, ever-more-complex mechanisms are developed for explaining the unacceptable while maintaining a façade of social and moral normality. Cohen's framework can help guide us through social responses to epidemic HIV/AIDS.

Giving Meaning to AIDS

From the very first days of the epidemic, AIDS was imbued with meaning. Driven equally by delight and disgust, conservative moralists rushed to declare that the virus manifested sin in all sorts of ways. People living with HIV and AIDS – and their partners and families – were marked out as sinful recipients of their just deserts from God. The epidemic itself was heralded as a harbinger of the apocalypse, a collective punishment from the Almighty, or a 'sin' against the cosmic order. Social scientists tend to dissect (and deride) arguments from sickness to sin because we do not recognize moral agency in an epidemic. Yet we may be at fault for neglecting what AIDS means for the moral universe and the power relations embedded therein.

Perhaps the most famous American exponent of AIDS as sin and punishment for sin was the Reverend Jerry Falwell, who in 1987 attributed the epidemic to divine retribution:

God says … that homosexuality is a perverted and reprobate lifestyle. God also says those engaged in such homosexual acts will receive 'in their own persons, due penalty of their error'. God destroyed Sodom and Gomorrah primarily because of the sin of homosexuality. Today, He is again bringing judgment against this wicked practice through AIDS.[7]

Falwell made similar comments about the terrorist crimes of 11 September 2001, pointing the finger at (among others) abortionists, homosexuals and the American Civil Liberties Union, on which occasion he was swiftly rebuked. In his apology, he blamed only the terrorists for the attacks but went on, 'I do believe, as a theologian, based upon many Scriptures and particularly Proverbs 14:23 [that] "living by God's principles promotes a nation to greatness, violating those principles brings a nation to shame".'[8] This parallel points us to how the AIDS pandemic is co-opted in service of a moral agenda and an imagination of apocalypse, as fascinating as it is terrifying. Fundamentalist moralists hold their hands over their eyes so as not to contemplate the sins they abhor, but cannot stop themselves peeking between their fingers.[9] Similarly we can rarely tell whether they fear or secretly relish the end of the world and the grotesque punishments in store for those who are not saved.

Frederic Chiluba, President of Zambia in the decade before the millennium (1991–2001), held similar views and even berated Peter Piot, Director of UNAIDS, on the subject.

Views not dissimilar to Falwell's and Chiluba's are expressed from an Islamist viewpoint by Malik Badri, a Sudanese psychiatrist and professor of Islamic civilization studies in Malaysia. He is one of the few Islamists to have written at length about HIV/AIDS:[10]

> The general [Muslim] belief about the AIDS pandemic is that of divine retribution for the immoral homosexual revolution of the West and its aping in other countries. This belief is firmly rooted in the Muslim mind because every child in his early school years must have been thrilled by the Qur'anic story of the Prophet Lot (pbuh [peace be upon him]) and what God did to his homosexual people [in Sodom and Gomorrah]. This is further ratified and explained in the most accurate and detailed exposition by a famous saying of the Prophet Muhammad (pbuh) in which he speaks as though he miraculously describes the contemporary dilemma of the AIDS pandemic. The famous *hadith* ... is translated as follows: 'If *fahashah* or fornication and all kinds of sinful sexual intercourse become *rampant and openly practised without inhibition* [emphasis in Badri] in any group or nation, Allah will punish them with *new epidemics (ta'un)* and new diseases which were not known to their forefathers and earlier generations.'

There are two reasons why Badri emphasizes sexual openness and lack of inhibition. Explicitly, he argues that an open community of practising homosexuals was essential for the emergence of a virulent strain of HIV.[11] Implicitly, Badri wishes to contrast the US gay subculture with the covert and private homosexuality of the Islamic world, which he does not mention in his book but could not deny. Badri goes on to speculate that God in His mercy destroyed Sodom and Gomorrah because a worse fate might have befallen its sinful inhabitants – AIDS. In turn he supposes that today's AIDS pandemic may be a mercifully dispatched deterrent to an even more terrible fate – public homosexuality.

As a practising psychiatrist, Dr Badri personally emphasizes the need for compassion and empathy with the individual living with HIV and AIDS – and he is careful to assert that they are victims rather than individual sinners or deviants. But he faithfully delineates the moral cosmology of political Islam and the place that AIDS occupies within it. Neo-fundamentalist preachers across the Muslim world are rather little preoccupied with AIDS – they have more tangible and immediate enemies to rail against – but their views are close to Badri's.

Christian and Muslim ethics and the AIDS epidemic are far more subtle than these examples might indicate. Marjorie Mbilinyi and Naomi Kaihula detail a vigorous local debate on the theology of AIDS in Rungwe, Tanzania.[12] Some religious leaders cannot wait for the Day of Judgment and are issuing verdict and sentence themselves. For example, in 1987 the Christian Council of Tanzania described AIDS as God's punishment for human beings' sins, and others have promoted 'a bitter, mean-spirited and punitive ideology … linking AIDS with transgression'.[13] Other Christians, however, have stressed forgiveness, repentance and faithfulness, while youth leaders have condemned the church for its hostility to condoms. The Jesuits have examined the AIDS pandemic with characteristic care and precision and conclude unequivocally that it is neither sin nor punishment, and that the doctrine of the lesser of two evils indicates that condoms should not always be condemned, and less harmful ways of drug use should be promoted.[14] The Catholic church, although late in responding to AIDS and profoundly compromised by papal opposition to condoms, has set up extremely extensive programmes of care and support to people affected by AIDS. Senegal's sufi clerics promote condoms, while Egypt has discreet helplines for women and men afraid of, or infected with HIV. Ugandan Muslim clerics declared 'jihad' against AIDS in 1989. Between condemnatory moralizing and enjoinders to share the burdens of the suffering are myriad moral positions too complex to be examined here.

The apocalyptic language of some religious moralizers might seem to dramatize AIDS's exceptional implications – the very reverse of denial. But closer examination suggests that the opposite happens. Those who preach in *extremis* moralizing about AIDS also peddle the same messages on other social ills (teenage pregnancy, drug abuse), natural disasters such as earthquakes, and terrorism – as illustrated by Falwell. For them, forecasting the end of the world is quite routine, and, as believers in the afterlife, they expect to be able to bask in glory when their prophecies of doom are proven right.[15] AIDS is normalized within their cosmos: it preserves and reinforces an existing moral order. Their congregations expect as much and are unlikely to show more fear or fervour over AIDS than when threatened with hurricanes or gay marriage.

'Normalizing' AIDS

The AIDS pandemic is a disaster with few parallels, because it is so easy to make it invisible or to pretend it is something else. An earthquake, flood or famine is dramatically visible and politically salient, because it affects entire communities in a spectacular fashion, including their leaders and spokespeople. AIDS is more like climate change, an incremental process manifest in a quickening drumbeat of 'normal' events. It is only by historic accident that epidemic HIV occurred within a few years of the scientific discovery of lenti-viruses[16] and the technologies that would make it possible to identify HIV at all. Had the pandemic struck a century earlier, it would have baffled even the most advanced microbiologists of the day and doubtless have fuelled the theories of those who ascribed disease to personal morality, the environment, or racial factors.

Where prevalence is low, the HIV/AIDS epidemic can readily be turned into an archipelago of isolated and 'normal' misfortunes. But where illness, bereavement and orphanhood are ubiquitous, effort and imagination are needed to pretend that everything is continuing as before and the moral world is intact. A person or society in denial would like to believe that life is perfectly normal, but in fact the thing that is being denied exerts a tremendous, if unacknowledged influence over every part of life. In anthropological terms, it is both taboo and totem. In Cohen's schema, the most sophisticated form of denial is 'normalization'. The intolerable becomes 'no longer news' and people invest in 'not having an inquiring mind about these matters'. Cohen further notes that private belief is less important than participating in the public affirmation of a lie.[17]

'Normalization' in the sense of adjusting reality to take account of the miseries of AIDS can be found in many places, when it is looked for. Even the statistics become numbing, and when lower-than-expected HIV prevalence is reported, as recently in Kenya and Zimbabwe, it can give the impression that things are 'not so bad' – when 7 or 10 per cent of an adult population is living with HIV. The study of socio-political denial is the study of how appearances are kept up, the moral order is sustained, and necessary changes are pressed into the service of existing interests. This can be seen at the family and community level, and in the way that national and international politics is managed.

In Botswana, Marguerite Daniel has studied orphans and the households that foster them and her detailed case studies show that people invest hugely in not changing.[18] The eldest of orphaned siblings may take on the role and title of 'father' or 'mother', or a foster carer may try to reproduce a 'normal' family, an effort which may at best draw a veil over the children's experiences and at worst draw them into abusive relationships with their caregivers. She describes the 'hidden wounds' of a society in denial, including the deep sadness of orphaned children, who are not told of their parents' illness and death, and often not even allowed to go to the funeral.

Daniel uses the concept of 'involution' to examine how communities continue functioning in the midst of so much death and trauma. 'Involution' refers to the short-term adaptations that an individual or community makes in the face of a serious threat which it cannot overcome. Central to these responses is clinging to the past and maintaining a reassuring familiarity. Over time, these stratagems become fixed and maladaptive, institutionalizing pervasive resistance to recognizing that HIV/AIDS demands some far-reaching changes in individual behaviour and social mores.

Daniel's account is the kind of fine-grained ethnography that is essential if we are to understand the scores of subtly different epidemics across Africa. It offers insights about Botswana that can be explored elsewhere. Her findings should not be taken as a general rule, just as different patterns in other countries cannot be said to refute her analysis. Above all, she shows that 'denial' is not a passive activity of failing to look, but an active task of struggling to maintain 'normality' when it is assaulted at every turn.

Sex and Power

Sex and gender are striking by their absence from the explicit social imaginary of AIDS. This is more surprising than it may seem, as power in Africa is accompanied by highly gendered imagery. Warmaking imagery – also a favoured vocabulary for the 'fight' against AIDS – is fiercely male. Rulers who have been in power for a few years are 'fathers' of their nations.[19] For Achille Mbembe, sexual domination is one of the symbolic and actual privileges of the ruler.[20] The subordinate position of women and girls – politically, socially and in sexual encounters – is ingrained in every aspect of the endemic. Although sex is rarely talked about publicly, sex acts are embedded in the most fundamental power relations and are symbolically represented in the imagery and ideological construction of the continent's big men.

Patriarchy is found in liberal and leftist political systems, too. Constituency-based electoral systems return a preponderance of men, often in proportion to how competitive they are. Leftist politics are deeply imbued with militarism and hegemonic masculinity. As Zimbabwean women insisted, 'Independence is not just for one sex.' Horace Campbell describes the phenomenon of 'Dodaism' which he calls a 'combination of patriarchal anxiety and deformed masculinity'.[21] This, he contends, underpins Robert Mugabe's homophobia, his pathological grip on power, and his ability to mobilize the anger of war veterans – real and imagined – in the pursuit of the fruits of victory which they feel they have been denied. Campbell argues that the liberationist left has yet to emancipate itself from an aggressive and regressive patriarchy.

The independence generation of African liberals and leftists shared traditionalists' aversion to dealing with sexuality and gender relations, and their legacy is still apparent. One of the key issues here is the sexual behaviour of many African men. The particular concern is that men often have one or more steady girlfriends in addition to their wives, and these girlfriends may have more than one regular boyfriend. Long-term concurrent sexual partnerships appear to be more common in sub-Saharan Africa than other parts of the world. Epidemiologists suspect a high level of such parallel partnerships is the key to why Africa has many HIV epidemics in the general population. The infect-ivity of a person living with HIV has two peaks. The first is shortly after becoming infected, as the virus multiplies and the immune system begins to respond. This lasts a few weeks, and is followed by a long period of many years in which infectivity is low and the chances of transmitting HIV during a single sexual contact are vanishingly small. Years later, when symptomatic AIDS develops, viral load increases and infectivity increases too, but by this time, sexual activity is likely to be reduced. Most onward transmission therefore occurs shortly after infection. Serial monogamy doesn't provide enough opportunities for this: only parallel partnerships will do. Commercial sex workers and their clients can easily be the focus for a concentrated epidemic. But if there are also many concurrent partnerships in the general population, then con-ditions are ripe for a generalized epidemic. The World Bank's *Confronting AIDS* includes an overview of this.[22] According to its summary, 'simulations show that HIV spreads most rapidly in populations with concurrent commercial, casual and marital sex, and least rapidly if there are no concurrent partnerships'.[23]

Several researchers have pursued this issue.[24] One is Helen Epstein. Her argument was not well-received in South Africa, where it was (mis)interpreted as another attempt by Western powers to condemn and control African sexuality. This was redolent of the angry debate over the 'African mode of sexuality' canvassed by the demographers John and Pat Caldwell.[25] In 1989 they argued that cultural values emphasizing female fertility, the high rate of concurrent sexual partnerships by men, and the fact that a significant number of women also had pre-marital or extra-marital sex, predisposed sub-Saharan Africa to a generalized heterosexual epidemic. The Caldwells were roundly criticized.[26] Their sources on African sexuality were often old, biased and unreliable. They overlooked the extent to which there is considerable social control – especially male control – over female sexuality. They were accused of reviving colonial era stereotypes of 'promiscuous natives' and of essentializing sexual cultures. This hostile response is understandable but it is unfortunate that it closed the door on open discussion of sexual networks.[27]

Investigating concurrency shines a light into the most intimate elements of human relationships. If concurrency is indeed the epidemiological key to southern Africa's AIDS epidemic, might it not also unlock another sociological puzzle, namely the explosion of sorcery accusations, widely observed and invariably attributed to jealousy (of which more later).

Another sexual reality that is commonly denied is homo-sexuality. Most Africans simply say 'it doesn't happen in our society'.[28] There is no gay voice in sub-Saharan African politics save in South Africa, where the ANC's coalition included gay rights activists.[29] However the leaders of the Gay Association of South Africa supported apartheid on the grounds that they didn't want to get involved in politics: 'they were just racists, homo-sexual racists'.[30] For its 'apolitical' stand – especially its failure to protest against the detention and trial for treason of one of its members, Simon Nkoli, for anti-apartheid activities in 1984 – GASA was suspended from the International Lesbian and Gay Association.

AIDS is failing to register in a critical zone of the public imagination. The silence over sex, gender and power is, in its way, a metaphor for the silence over AIDS. It can be seen, within Cohen's schematization, as a case of 'interpretative denial': the existence of AIDS is acknowledged, but the implication that one might need to change one's personal beliefs and behaviour is not.

Domesticating AIDS – and Its Costs

An epidemic such as AIDS disturbs the moral order. Christians and Muslims wrestle with the problem of a loving/merciful God sending a lethal infection. Traditional belief systems and moral frameworks are ubiquitous in Africa, overlapping with Muslim and Christian faith, and uniting the socio-political realm and the world of spiritual powers.[31] These beliefs lack professional exponents, obliging us to turn to social anthropologists for interpretation. Again, we see communities and individuals paying a high price for society's hard work in reconstructing 'normality' amidst AIDS.

In *Witchcraft, Violence and Democracy in South Africa*,[32] Adam Ashforth asks why sorcery accusations have become so much more common in Soweto since the end of apartheid. He describes a 'presumption of malice' in community life,[33] how accusations of witchcraft arise from personal jealousies and community tensions, and the way in which supernatural claims are compatible with scientific thinking. If everyday physics explains *how* things happen, only witchcraft can explain *why* something happens to an individual on a particular occasion, in a world where nothing is presumed to happen by accident alone. This is ethnography in the classic tradition of Edward Evans-Pritchard's studies among the Azande of Southern Sudan.[34] Alongside sorcerers, the main wielders of invisible power are ancestor spirits, whose authority provides stability to a collective moral and social order. Individual spirits can support or torment the living, depending on the circumstances in which they died and the manner in which their continuing needs are met – or not.[35]

Soweto residents attribute powers to the invisible world in a very literal manner which can take by surprise those – such as secular academics – living what Ashforth calls 'bleakly sub-monotheistic lives'. Christian missionaries' worldviews are more compatible. One Colorado evangelist wrote a report entitled 'Towards the Spiritual Mapping of Dobsonville, Soweto', which tabulated the levels, types and significance of demonic activity. While Sowetans might disagree with the churchman's labels for the spiritual forces at work, they would have no difficulty with the exercise in cataloguing those powers.

Throughout the 1990s, life in Soweto remained hard, and it was no longer possible to attribute misfortune to the apartheid authorities. Suffering lost its meaning. Sowetans' spirit-scape is further imperilled by the AIDS epidemic, particularly by the number of early and 'bad' deaths it entails. As Ashforth notes, living to the Biblical three score years and ten is now a 'privilege' enjoyed by few,[36] the funerals of adults who have died of AIDS are routine, and the virus and disease remain subject to many taboos. Elevation to ancestorhood is straightforward if one passes away at a ripe old age, with lifetime obligations completed, surrounded by children and grandchildren. Such a person becomes readily integrated into the web of collective ancestral authority and may become posthumously recognized as the founder of a lineage. By contrast, someone who dies early of a disfiguring and dishonourable disease – especially with few or no offspring – is likely to be a disturbed and disturbing ancestral spirit. As the authority of ancestors is the basis for kinship organization and the main regulator of family harmony, this profusion of discontented spirits spells trouble for the social sphere.

An investigation by Christopher Desmond and his colleagues in Swaziland,[37] a country in which two thirds of the population live on less than a dollar a day, found that the average cost of a funeral was in the range US$473–US$704, with only a modest decrease noted between 1998 and 2002. Costs include keeping the body in the morgue until the burial can be organized, purchase of coffin and gravesite, announcements on the radio and in the newspapers, transport of the body, widow's garments, and the provision of substantial amounts of food for the numerous funeral guests. Some families, there is no doubt, bury their dead in painfully simple circumstances. But, for the majority, it all adds up to a formidable expense and often a crippling financial strain. Some administrators and chiefs have tried to limit the expense of funerals, but with little success. As Desmond and his colleagues note:

Observations relating to burial practices in Swaziland have shown very little evidence of practices adapting to a changing environment. Although undertakers have shown a response to the increasing numbers of AIDS-related deaths in keeping their prices constant despite inflation, burial practices do not reflect any change. One could speculate that cultural beliefs and practices are a strong force in opposing change, yet the ritual of large and expensive funerals is itself only fairly recent and not an established custom.[38]

At a Swazi funeral, AIDS will almost never be mentioned. Every effort will be made to maintain a veneer of normality. Desmond and his colleagues attribute this to denial. This deserves further examination. Insisting on 'normality' in funerals serves to retain faith in a cosmic normality. The more the deceased is handicapped in achieving benevolent ancestorhood, the greater the efforts that need to be made on her or his behalf by the surviving relatives. An elaborate funeral is an investment of earthly resources to maintain the invisible order. This phenomenon began and continues independently of AIDS – Africa's most elaborate funerals are found in coastal West African countries where the epidemic has been less devastating – but AIDS has become totemic for this cosmological crisis.

The Gwembe Tonga communities of rural Zambia have been studied by anthropologists for half a century. They report a marked increase in sorcery accusations and also a long-term increase in funeral costs.[39] As in Soweto, jealousies drive witchcraft allegations often among intimate kin.

What, indeed, can a society do when threatened by an invisible enemy, which is destroying the life chances of an entire generation? Catherine Campbell's *Letting Them Die: Why HIV/AIDS Programmes Fail*[40] is another superb ethnography of contemporary South African township life. It focuses on how mineworkers, commercial sex workers and other residents of the pseudonymous

'Summertown' are locked into belief systems, behavioural patterns and economic constraints that condemn them to a very high risk of contracting HIV and dying of AIDS. Campbell is a social psychologist and her account is framed accordingly: what she describes are personal cosmologies. The world of the men who labour underground is marked by a very high perceived risk of accidents at work, and an emotionally impoverished life in single-sex workers' hostels. Theirs is a risky life, their masculine identities given meaning by the fact that they face perils underground each day. Avoiding risk during sexual encounters has little meaning. Meanwhile their craving for intimacy is symbolized by skin-on-skin sex, which is a personal liberty central to their sense of self, not just an epidemiological bad habit. For the women, all poor and competing in an over-supplied market for sexual services, the 'choice' of unprotected sex is simply a financial trade-off between less money today (and the threat of physical violence from a dissatisfied client) and the far-off danger of developing AIDS. This has echoes, too, of the risk of a 'bad reputation' weighed by women in Kampala who too rarely insist on condom use to protect themselves.[41]

In Campbell's Summertown, as in Soweto, without a miracle cure, universal antiretroviral treatment or an equally miraculous social and behavioural revolution, well over half of today's teen-agers will die of AIDS, most of them in their late twenties or thirties. Yet at the time of Campbell's research, AIDS was still an unspoken taboo. In a world saturated with unmanageable risk, it was too much to contemplate. Ashforth comes to a similar con-clusion. The spiritual insecurity experienced by Sowetans, he argues, has clear implications for public safety. It is fuelling much local violence. The difficulty is that witchcraft belongs to 'a different realm of action and experience from politics, something personal, speculative, and open-ended'[42] in contrast to the reper-toire of political issues and ideologies familiar to anyone involved in the struggle against apartheid. If spiritual forces operate in a different sphere to the rule of law and human rights, then democratic politics is failing to deal with a fundamental problem in people's lives and after-lives.

The repercussions of AIDS for the moral cosmology are profound indeed. The secular frameworks of epidemiology and public policy will not by themselves be enough to make sense of the virus and epidemic. We need to develop and deploy metaphors that speak to the social world, constructed around moral imaginings which are impacted by AIDS and which in turn constrain social capabilities to respond to AIDS. We should also be alert to the fact that scholars and policy makers themselves are unable to think about the crisis that is AIDS without using language and imagery borrowed from another realm of human experience. How we think about the AIDS epidemic becomes its own reality.

Yet we must not lose sight of the virus and the disease. Susan Sontag has warned of the perils of clothing illness in metaphor.[43] The evolutionary theorist Stephen Jay Gould is an exemplar of the scientific objective approach: 'AIDS represents the ordinary workings of biology, not an irrational or diabolical plague with moral meaning.'[44] HIV transmission is preventable and medication is available that can extend a healthy life for those living with HIV. Science can triumph, given resources, policies and the right social and political context. Our metaphors and models are not fixed: they can become truer to reality, and thereby hold the potential for changing reality. And there is some evidence that this is happening.

The Media and Overcoming Denial

African publics are becoming more concerned about AIDS as a public policy issue. Afrobarometer surveys show a low but increasing number of respondents mentioning AIDS as a problem warranting government action. We have seen that this increased concern is not mainly driven by personal experience. The Afro-barometer data allow us to identify what is bringing about this change. The most prominent factors are the individual's level of education and how often he or she reads a newspaper.[45] In a study prepared for this book, Jacob Bor has analysed the data further, comparing fourteen countries. His most powerful finding is that three country-level indicators – national HIV prevalence, level of radio access, and the freedom of the press – explain almost all of the variation in the percentage of respondents recognizing HIV/AIDS as a problem deserving government action. An astonishing 92 per cent of the country-level variation is explained by just these three factors. Moreover, these factors far outweigh 'reported personal loss due to AIDS' in explaining why some individuals prioritize AIDS and others do not.[46] Most important are the overall levels of media access and quality in a country.

Furthermore, Bor finds a robust positive correlation between the freedom of the press (measured using Freedom House rankings) and 'political commitment' in AIDS programme effort.[47] More than any other political factor measured, a free press is positively associated with energetic governmental AIDS policies.

Communication through the media appears to be the key in overcoming denial and turning recognition of the AIDS epidemic into determination to make it a policy priority. But it is not simple. It is not that public education messages are getting through in some places and not others. The pathway is much more interesting than that, and can be fleshed out with careful analysis of how AIDS is handled in the media.

In a study prepared for this book, Charles Wendo has analysed the Ugandan media and how it portrays AIDS, and has meshed this analysis with what is known about popular attitudes to the disease in that country.[48] The overwhelming majority of Ugandans – well over 90 per cent, and more women than men – think that AIDS is a legitimate topic for the media. The newspapers and radio run AIDS news stories frequently. Most people's beliefs about AIDS, however, are shaped by their *personal* interactions with friends and family members. Ugandan society is characterized by a high level of everyday informal discussion about AIDS, which seems to have been critically important in driving ordinary people's behavioural change. The media's role is important but indirect. Radio and newspapers are bad at influencing what people think, but news stories are good at setting the topics that people talk about.

Wendo's analysis provides us with the following pathway. The first step is the creation of 'news'. What counts as 'news' is determined by a fairly small set of opinion formers, including government officials, international aid officials, scientists, doctors and activists. Most newspaper stories are generated by official announcements and events, such as international conferences, the inauguration of projects, or the publication of statistics on World AIDS Day every December. These stories – especially those of international provenance – get more space than scientific reports about risks of infection and possibilities for treatment. Most readers prefer to place their trust in doctors and people with professional credentials.

The second step is for the newspapers to pick up these stories, particularly the two up-market English language dailies, the *New Vision* (government-owned but with a fair degree of editorial independence) and the *Monitor* (a private newspaper). Although read by a relatively small number of urbanites, the papers set the tone for news about AIDS. The quality and credibility of the newspapers are the key to their role, not the size of their readership. If they report well on the full complexity of the issue, they are more likely to be believed by their readers.

The next step is the translation of quality into reach. Among those readers are the news and feature editors of Uganda's numerous radio stations. In deciding what to schedule for radio programming that day, the radio editors pick the morning's most

interesting newspaper articles. The better the quality of newspaper reporting, the more likely the radio stations are to run the
story. Official and independent radio news editors make similar
decisions. FM radio stations are most listened to in the towns and
along major transport arteries, and government broadcasts in the
rural areas. The reach of the radio now becomes important: most
Ugandans obtain their news from radio. And far more people
listen to the news than to public service announcements and educational messages.

Fourth, in turn, the news stories and on-air discussions set the
agenda for what people discuss at home, in public transport, in
bars and at other social events. Public service and educational
announcements do not count for much – even if people listen to
them, they tend to discount them. But while exhortations and
similar messages are filtered out, news stories set people talking.
Listeners are sceptical enough to dispute what they hear and
disagree with any advice proffered, but they discuss, and these
interpersonal discussions are the situation in which people learn
from one another and forge opinions. Curiously, if this analysis is
correct, then it is actually counterproductive for all AIDS advocates
to be 'on message', because that makes people bored, sceptical
and switched-off. Having been fed propaganda for decades they
are instinctively distrustful of any message purveyed with earnest
consensus. On the contrary, African radio listeners are not so
naïve as to be confused by uncertainty and debate. Rather, there
should be vigorous debates about what is actually correct,
including voicing dissident or denialist positions – to encourage
people to discuss.

The major difficulty facing journalists and editors is that the
AIDS 'story' rarely changes. Far more people are killed by HIV
than by criminals, but every crime is different, while most cases
of AIDS are depressingly similar – and people do not want to talk
much about the personal circumstances or medical details that
distinguish one from another. This makes it hard for reporters to

find a new angle on AIDS, as a result of which there are few stories initiated by the journalists themselves. The newspapers cover about one AIDS story per paper per day, and these mostly consist of reporting on AIDS-related events such as donors giving funds, or workshops and conferences on the topic. On balance, AIDS is reported as a 'positive' or 'good news' story: the news usually focuses on events such as funds being donated and projects opening. Wendo quotes the *New Vision* news editor John Baptist Wasswa's explanation for this: 'People have suffered so much and you don't want to frustrate the reader by giving them more bad news than good news. It also makes business sense because people are more likely to read the paper if there is hope in the story.'[49]

Politicians and administrators have the most regular profile in AIDS stories in the Ugandan press. Medical specialists and researchers are cited less often. There are fewer stories about international agencies and donors, but when the papers run them, they are given more space and may get front-page billing. The message is consistent to the point of being formulaic. It may not be exciting but it keeps AIDS in the news. Such coverage may risk dampening interpersonal discussions, however, because it is too dull. Interestingly, readers demand more medical and scientific stories, and less coverage of politicians and programmes. People want the facts, debates and news.

Ugandans are sophisticated consumers of news. With a diet of 'good news' stories and a decreasing rate of HIV, we might expect the Ugandan public to be enthusiastic about its government's much-lauded HIV/AIDS efforts. Afrobarometer data show that public response is more complicated.[50] Opinion is split down the middle. While most Ugandans view the government's actions favourably, the substantial minority who want more attention to AIDS do not think that the government is doing a good enough job. Perhaps, after the high-profile government AIDS campaigns of the late 1980s, Ugandans may think that their leaders have let

the issue slip. Or they may not believe that the credit for the
country's success should go to the government, preferring to
attribute success to civil society. Or they may be sceptical of the
claim that AIDS is actually in retreat.

Pavement Radio

The missing piece in this argument is exactly what kind of discussions are sparked by news about AIDS. No researcher has
investigated what people actually talk about, as opposed to how
they receive official educational messages. We can, however,
approach this question indirectly, through those professional
observers of everyday life: novelists. A small sample of African
novels in English provides a first cut at exploring this topic, and it
is clear that AIDS is approached indirectly, in diverse ways,
through other issues.

In *Far and Beyon'*, Unity Dow describes the level of sexual
harassment and predation faced by schoolgirls in Botswana, and
the continuing public silence and shame over 'this disease' and
those who 'die of a long illness'.[51] Neshani Andreas tells of how a
man's death in a Namibian village is attributed to the sorcery of
jealous relatives, and is followed by poisonous recriminations
and greedy dispossession, leaving the widow destitute.[52] Both
these tales conclude with the triumph of female solidarity.
Phaswane Mpe's *Welcome to Our Hillbrow* is a more urban and edgy
story.[53] It opens with the fatal violence of the residents of the
Johannesburg neighbourhood as they cheer a football victory,
spinning cars in the street and hurling bottles from balcony
windows. A little girl is knocked down and killed. The risks of
AIDS are embedded within the dangers of crime and celebration.
In this mixed and vibrant community, still hung over from the
apartheid years in which morality was reduced to skill in deploy-
ing euphemism, HIV is attributed to *makwerekwere* – itinerants,

sojourners, sex workers and foreigners, the latter mostly Niger-
ians and Zairois. It is a disease from somewhere else – specifically
identified with people who are thought to be troublemakers. But
the narrator quickly points out that 'there are very few Hill-
browans, if you think about it, who were not originally wanderers
from Tiragolong and other rural villages, who have come here, as
we have, in search of education and work. Many of the
Makwerekwere you accuse of this and that are no different to us....'[54]

Although AIDS is central to these stories, it is rarely mentioned
as such. The focus is on the social and personal problems that the
epidemic generates, and how people deal with those. Politics is
present: the politics of relations between the sexes and the generations, between residents and newcomers. The government
barely figures. The official representatives of the health establishment, including HIV testing centres, are problematic places that
people approach with trepidation. These novels illuminate how
apparent silence can be conjoined with recognition of the
problem of AIDS, expressed at a different level. There are
unexplored agendas here for journalists.

Africans are hungry for real news about AIDS and the debates
swirling around it. People want to be kept informed about medical,
epidemiological and scientific news, which they will then discuss
and assess. Dealing with the personal, family and communal
impacts is another important topic. High-quality news, analysis
and opinion appear to be the best way of breaking down denial,
weakening the grip of moral and cosmic metaphor, and promoting public commitment to tackling AIDS. How an informed
citizenry then articulates and enforces its demands is a different
question.

3

AIDS Activists: Reformers and Revolutionaries

Confrontation and Its Limits

On 12 July 2005, demonstrators from the Treatment Action Campaign (TAC) occupied the hospital in Queenstown in the Eastern Cape Province of South Africa to deliver a memorandum to the provincial health administrators. The demonstration ended with police opening fire. Seventy-six foreign development and AIDS organizations including UNAIDS condemned the police brutality, and the AIDS Healthcare Foundation expressed its outrage over 'the first-ever police shooting of AIDS protesters anywhere worldwide'.[1] From a continent away this looked like a life-and-death confrontation between desperate AIDS patients and an uncaring government with a conspicuously bad AIDS policy, possibly the harbinger of riots and revolution. It wasn't. Part of the reason is that AIDS activism is not a revolutionary political project.

As South African protests go, the Queenstown sit-in was unexceptional – there are almost daily demonstrations against unemployment and local government cutting off water or electricity supplies, which are marked by street rallies, burning tyres, and provocations to the local police. Exactly how many demonstrators entered the hospital, how much they disrupted activities there, and for how long, is uncertain from contradictory media accounts. What is clear is that they did not leave when the hospital authorities asked. The police bungled the job of removing them, firing teargas and rounds of rubber bullets, injuring ten. No live ammunition was fired. Another thirty demonstrators suffered from beating and trampling. One was admitted to the hospital and kept overnight while another needed stitches.

Had this been a protest by the United Democratic Front twenty years earlier, at the height of the confrontation with the apartheid government, the injured would have been celebrities in the struggle. Violent clashes would have ratcheted up. That didn't happen after Queenstown: the TAC condemned the violence but didn't use it to escalate confrontation, let alone challenge the legitimacy of President Thabo Mbeki and his African National Congress government – despite Mbeki's bizarre and harmful public statements that HIV does not cause AIDS. The TAC statement concluded:

> TAC will mobilize a mass demonstration in Queenstown on 26 July 2005. We ask all civil society organizations and individuals to join us in this protest against unnecessary HIV deaths, for treatment and against police brutality. We will march to enforce our constitutional rights to life, dignity, freedom to demonstrate, equality and access to health care....The TAC NEC [National Executive Committee] salutes our Queenstown and Eastern Cape comrades. We say to our leaders in the Eastern Cape: we are proud of your work – mobilize to ensure at least 200,000 [people get treatment] by 2006 and that ultimately everyone who needs treatment gets it.[2]

There is a real political struggle over AIDS and AIDS treatment in South Africa, but it is totally different from the fight to bring down apartheid. The TAC uses some of the same language of people's struggle, because that is South Africa's language of politics.

But – as some Eastern Cape leaders were quick to point out – many of the TAC protesters were themselves loyal ANC members. For the TAC leadership, the ANC, despite its errors, is still the people's government.

The TAC is distinctively South African and needs to be seen in the very specific context of that country's unique history, or it will be easy to draw the wrong conclusions. The TAC is not an opposition party seeking to destabilize or bring down the government. On many issues it is in fact sympathetic to the ruling ANC; indeed, it supported the government in its legal action against international pharmaceutical companies to allow for the import and production of cheaper generic medicines. Its civil disobedience campaigns are aimed at enforcing the rights enshrined in South Africa's constitution.[3] Despite its name, the TAC is not a single-issue campaign. Neither, despite its 'HIV Positive' T-shirts, is it a vehicle for the identity politics of people living with HIV and AIDS.

South Africans tend to see political and social life through the lens of apartheid and the struggle against it. The TAC is a step-child of the popular struggle that brought racist rule to an end. The United Democratic Front was the legal face of opposition during the later apartheid years, utilizing non-violent methods of political activism that included strikes and demonstrations. While never ceding the legitimacy of the apartheid government, UDF activists used the law to challenge every aspect of racist and arbitrary rule. UDF members were backed by a three-cornered coalition comprising the ANC, the Congress of South African Trade Unions (COSATU) and the South African Communist Party (SACP). The ANC, with its military wing Umkhonto we Sizwe, sought to make the country ungovernable and renounced violence only when progress at the Conference for a Democratic South Africa made a non-racial democracy inevitable.

The TAC was created in 1998 by individuals who had been active in the UDF, including members of the ANC. Zackie Achmat and Mark Heywood were prominent among them. Many of the methods of struggle are familiar from the old days of the struggle against apartheid, including civil disobedience campaigns, public rallies, citizens' education and the use of the courts to challenge executive decisions. The best-known court-based challenge was the effort to make the South African government commit itself to providing nevirapine to prevent mother-to-child transmission of HIV. They even took the melodies of ANC-UDF songs and changed the lyrics. The core organizational principles reflect the founders' schooling in Leninist forms of covert mobilization: a dedicated, close-knit vanguard at the centre of a broad front. As well as a membership of over 10,000 – a vocal minority of the five million South Africans living with HIV and AIDS – the TAC has entered into its own tripartite coalition with COSATU and the SACP. The targets of its activism, like those of its precursor, include not only the South African government but also Western governments and international companies.

Zackie Achmat explains how TAC leaders 'had to transform the old slogan: "Mobilize! Don't Mourn" into "Mobilize and Mourn." We had to learn law, epidemiology, science, mathematics, medicine, pharmacology, ethics, political economy, and international relations.' The result has been that 'thousands of TAC members living in poverty-stricken conditions with limited educational backgrounds are capable of explaining how nevirapine or other antiretroviral medicines prevents mother-to-child transmission. So can many other South Africans as a result of the public information campaigns that the TAC ran.'[4]

But South Africa today is completely changed from the 1980s and 1990s. The TAC has no agenda of overthrowing the government or denying its legitimacy. Many remain as members of the ANC. Not only do they have personal friends and comrades within the party and government, but they are very sympathetic to many of the policies of the Mbeki government. It is their government and constitution; they are still proud of both.

In its early years, the TAC fashioned itself as a single-issue campaign focusing on government provision of antiretrovirals, along with efforts to break the stigma surrounding infection with HIV. It still does these things and has brought personal salvation to many people living with HIV and AIDS who were isolated and depressed. But, especially after the government ceded the principle of universal antiretroviral treatment (ART) in 2003, it has positioned itself as part of a wider struggle for social and economic rights in South Africa.

Many South Africans, including trade unionists and communists, are highly critical of the economic policies of the ANC since it was elected, arguing that promises of major improvements in health, education and utilities such as water and electricity have been betrayed. But the critique is as sympathetic as it is adversarial: the ANC's challengers recognize that the government is operating under tight constraints.

The TAC was careful to campaign for universal ART only when the price of drugs had fallen in 2002–3. Until then, the leaders knew that the price was so prohibitive that universal provision would have spelled national bankruptcy, and they were not prepared to campaign for that. The campaign has parallels and links with a host of other social movements in South Africa focusing on land rights, a 'people's budget', electricity provision, education, transport and a basic income grant.[5] Today, the TAC leaders insist that AIDS treatment should be part of a broad package of social and economic rights including food, shelter and employment. This is more than tactical deference to its allies' concerns. They see that AIDS can be overcome only with wide-ranging social and economic emancipation and they are well-attuned to how South Africans think about politics.

At a June 2005 TAC youth march in Kayelitsha, banners read, '1976: Youth against Apartheid. 2002: Youth against HIV/AIDS'. (It was a recycled old banner.) The adversary was the disease, not the government. Other banners read, 'Food, ARVs [antiretrovirals],

Health for All'. TAC has forged an alliance with COSATU, the SACP, the South African Council of Churches and other groups in the Save Jobs Coalition. In doing so, it has tapped into the political contract that COSATU and the SACP have with the ANC in government. TAC joined COSATU for a strike and rally in Cape Town on 27 June 2005. When Zackie mounted the podium for his brief speech to the crowd, he did not mention AIDS once. Many other speakers had mentioned AIDS as one of the issues demanding action. Zackie stressed solidarity for social justice.

The TAC leadership has taken great care over how it frames AIDS as a political issue. While its legal and organizational energies are directed to treatment access, its political rhetoric places AIDS within broader social and economic rights. It wants to change government policy, not the government. It seeks to realize the social and economic rights enshrined in the constitution through a mixture of legal activism and public protest. This approach is reflected in South African public opinion. South Africans are critical of their government's policies and think more should be done about AIDS. But they don't want AIDS to be prioritized at the expense of other pressing social and economic issues. More than any other country, South Africans reject the notion that AIDS should be sacrificed for development – or development for AIDS.

Has TAC influenced public opinion or has it designed its campaign to tap into existing political currents? Undoubtedly both propositions are true. The end result is a political challenge to the ANC. The challenge is fundamental in the sense that it demands that the ANC return to its older philosophy of being a people's movement for social change as well as a political party. It is less so, in that it seeks this change from within. The TAC's accommodation to the ruling party is strategic, because the ANC is likely to be in power for a long time. It is consistent, because the TAC is still broadly sympathetic to its former comrades-in-arms. It is also consonant with the dominant idioms of African politics, which stress consensus not confrontation.

'Positive Positive Women'

The TAC is the most visible of Africa's AIDS activist organizations. But much more common is a welfare-focused approach that amalgamates community mobilization for care giving and education with channelling foreign project funding. This is driven by a combination of personal exposure to the disease and its effects, a ready-to-hand model for responding (the 'local NGO') and the availability of donor funds for these activities. A growing number of volunteers and activists, overwhelmingly women, work as counsellors, care givers and local advocates for change. Often, learning their or their partner's HIV status was the spark for activism. Richard Dowden calls them the 'positive positive women'.

> Such a person is Siphiwe Hlophe who had just turned forty in 1999 when she won a scholarship to study agricultural economics in Britain. She has four children, the eldest 22 years old, and the youngest eleven. One of the conditions of the scholarship was an AIDS test, which she took not thinking there was a problem. She turned out to be HIV-positive. Her husband left her, she lost her scholarship and she thought she was going to die. Then she decided to do something for people living with AIDS. She formed a group called SWAPOL, Swaziland for Positive Living, made up of mostly HIV-positive women. It now has 150 members. They walk and talk and sing with the swagger of conquerors, visiting terminally ill people in their homes, ensuring they get medical care and a healthy diet. Mrs Hlophe laughs. 'We are so busy. Now I'm going to live to my retirement.'

Siphiwe's experience echoes that of Noerine Kaleeba, who founded The AIDS Support Organization (TASO) in Uganda in 1987, after her husband Christopher was diagnosed with AIDS while studying in England.[6] Noerine herself is HIV-negative, but twelve of her co-founders of TASO were living with HIV and

AIDS. A physiotherapist by background, Noerine had worked with disabled people and had observed how they suffered stigma and discrimination from the community. But she was shocked by the level of fear and aversion expressed towards AIDS – not just by ordinary people, but also by health workers. When Christopher had been hospitalized in England, the nurses had given him good care and support – despite the fact that he was the only black patient in a large provincial hospital. In Mulago, Uganda's flagship hospital, Noerine reports that the nurses were afraid even to touch Christopher. He died shortly after returning to Uganda.

TASO began with just fifteen volunteers and grew to be a nationwide organization serving 65,000 people. From the outset, it suffered both the grief and the warmth that have been characteristics of pioneering efforts in the field of AIDS. Twelve of the founders died of AIDS within the first year. But hundreds more who had at first scorned the organization, and shared the fear and revulsion, changed their views. Many of them did so as their own friends and relatives fell sick with AIDS.

For fifteen years after TASO was founded – until ART became widely available – organizations run by people living with HIV and AIDS suffered dreadful losses. Other NGOs also saw their staff ebbing away – if not sick, then perhaps drawn out of work to help care for someone ill with AIDS, or for orphans. This horrible attrition rate could point to another explanation for public indifference: those who care are dying, becoming exhausted, or withdrawing from public life.

There is some evidence for this. In 2002, Ryann Manning of the Health Economics and HIV/AIDS Research Division of the University of KwaZulu-Natal investigated the impact of AIDS on a spectrum of NGOs in that province. Of the 59 community-based organizations she surveyed, 76 per cent reported that HIV/AIDS was already impacting on their organization and their work, though in most cases not yet severely. She reported, 'The strongest finding to come out of this research, consequently, was not about the current impact, but rather the inevitable and imminent future one.'[7]

AIDS is putting stresses on voluntary organizations and there are fears that it undermines community life. In some places this may be happening – for example, Afrobarometer data imply that Mozambicans who provide home-based care are less likely to attend rallies and protests or discuss politics. But AIDS is also the reason why many such organizations have been created, and in many countries – Tanzania, Mali and South Africa among them – people involved in home-based care are also more likely to be politically active. From the survey data, we cannot say if care giving makes people more politically engaged, or if those who are more politically active are impelled to become carers. But, either way, we can concur with Samantha Willan's observation from South Africa: 'AIDS has created a "pillar" to organize around, and in the process has led to new organizations forming and strengthened old ones.'[8] She sees pockets of community mobilization: many grandmothers are responding to the increasing needs and are caring for the grandchildren and the sick; many have formed sewing groups and support groups, and are starting vegetable gardens to feed those in need. Similarly, youth groups are forming for AIDS awareness and education campaigns. Most notably, treatment and care have become a focus for energy, both to lobby the government for policy change, and also to assist with treatment literacy, fighting stigma, promoting testing, and ensuring that people access, and then adhere to, treatment regimes.

AIDS and Elections

Citizens in African democracies do not recognize AIDS as their top concern, and Africa's leading AIDS activists are careful not to challenge their government's legitimacy on the issue. It follows that AIDS will not head elected politicians' agendas either, no matter how much foreign AIDS ambassadors try to persuade them otherwise. This helps explain why the response of African governments to HIV/AIDS has been rather limited.

This may also help explain Jacob Bor's striking and counter-intuitive finding: that the leaders of democratic countries have exhibited no more political commitment to AIDS than more autocratic rulers.[9] Bor correlated Freedom House 'political rights' scores, a measure of electoral accountability, and AIDS Program Effort Index 'political support' scores, while accounting for rival hypotheses. His findings confound the expectation that electoral democracy is automatically good for AIDS effort. Press freedom had a consistently positive association with political support for AIDS policies. Controlling for this, among high-prevalence countries, the relationship between electoral accountability and political support for AIDS policies was robustly if modestly negative.

The story is different in different countries. Per Strand has extracted four different kinds of 'AIDS constituencies' from the Afrobarometer data.[10] The 'critical constituency' thinks AIDS is an important issue, that the government isn't handling it well, and that it should be given greater priority in public policy. The 'ambiguous' constituency agrees with one or two of those propositions. The 'positive constituency' thinks that AIDS is a priority and the government is doing well. Where there are no strong views, there is no AIDS constituency.

Botswana is a unique example of a strong 'positive constituency'. It has the highest level of public confidence in government policy on AIDS, strongly correlated with demand for public action on AIDS. This implies that the government is successfully setting the nation's AIDS agenda. But some Batswana also feel that the government has done all it can on AIDS and should not lose focus on other public issues. In South Africa, Namibia and Uganda, the 'critical constituency' dominates: an independent civil society leads the national debate on AIDS, and citizens are demanding that the government do more. This is unsurprising in South Africa because of Thabo Mbeki's denialist position, but less expected in Uganda. In a number of countries – Ghana, Mali, Mozambique, Tanzania and Zambia – there is no evident AIDS constituency at all.

African electors' low level of political concern over AIDS also allows us to explain why the ANC seems unhurt electorally by Thabo Mbeki's stand on HIV/AIDS. Mbeki has publicly adopted the extreme view that HIV is not the cause of AIDS and that anti-retroviral treatment is unnecessary and toxic. A bizarre episode in South African history and Mbeki's own career, this has been an immense impediment to a sensible HIV/AIDS policy in South Africa. Given the scale of the country's AIDS crisis, its democratic electoral system and free press, this would appear to spell political disaster. If he were presiding over the starvation of a quarter of South African citizens there seems little doubt that Mbeki would be voted out of office. South Africans went to the polls in April 2004. Samantha Willan analysed the election results with an eye to the impact of HIV/AIDS.[11] It cannot be discerned. The most striking outcome is that the ANC achieved an overwhelming majority of support, with almost 70 per cent of the vote, and won control of all nine provinces, including the Western Cape and KwaZulu-Natal, previously held by opposition parties or in coalition with the ANC.

In the run-up to South Africa's first democratic election in 1994, Nelson Mandela was reportedly advised not to make AIDS into a campaign issue for fear of offending culturally conservative constituencies. 'I wanted to win,' said Mandela, 'and I did not talk about AIDS.'[12]

During Thabo Mbeki's first term as President (1999–2004), AIDS became an issue of public controversy. Mbeki's personal denialist position generated widespread criticism – and possibly gave the issue of HIV/AIDS more public visibility than if he had quietly gone along with the international consensus. The survey conducted by Afrobarometer in 2002 reports that for the question on 'government performance on AIDS' the South African government earned the lowest rating of all countries surveyed: just 30 per cent responded 'fairly well', and 15 per cent 'very well'.[13] This dissatisfaction was expressed through TAC protests, through the media, and through a chorus of international dismay.

The prospect of the 2004 election seems to have pushed Mbeki to shift his position. In the middle of 2003, he started taking a lower public profile on AIDS – leading some to speculate that he might have changed his mind (he hadn't). The party began to promise expanded AIDS treatment, and also changed its language on HIV/AIDS towards considering the options of treatment and care. The first target announced was to have 53,000 people on treatment by 31 March 2004[14] – a date suspiciously close to voting day. The target was not met: by the end of June 2004 the TAC estimated that fewer than 10,000 South Africans were on public sector treatment,[15] and the government extended its deadline for reaching 53,000 by a further twelve months. It was too little and too late. Official government estimates are that fully 500,000 South Africans needed treatment.

The President's State of the Nation speech in February 2004 lacked any sense of urgency over AIDS. The epidemic was mentioned in passing as one of the challenges, but without emphasis.[16] After the election, President Mbeki's inaugural speech on 27 April again failed to mention HIV/AIDS in a meaningful way. AIDS appears to have mattered enough to make the government adjust its course, but not enough to make it reverse direction. Mbeki read the political mood correctly, and it didn't change the electoral result. Zackie read the political mood equally astutely. TAC did not call on its members to boycott the election or vote against ANC candidates. And this was not just a tactical decision: it reflected the TAC's strategy and philosophy of changing policies, not governments.

Activist Networks, Local and Global

American AIDS activist Larry Kramer began a 1983 article entitled '1,112 and Counting' with the words, 'If this article doesn't scare the shit out of you, we're in real trouble. If this article doesn't rouse you to anger, fury, rage, and action, gay men may have no future on this earth. Our continued existence depends on just how angry you can get.'[17] Kramer's activism began on the North American fringes, framed by the identity politics of the gay community and in enraged opposition to a Republican administration that it saw as at best callous, at worst genocidal.[18] He and other American (including African-American) writers and advocates used 'genocide' and 'holocaust' to describe AIDS's march of death.[19] The theme recurs in different guises, including 'genocide' by impact if not intent, or as wilful neglect of certain populations (gays, black people[20]) whom the authorities would happily see die off.[21]

African AIDS activism began at the fringes also. The first activists in Uganda – the singer Philly Lutaaya, Bishop Misaeri Kauma and Noerine Kaleeba – were encouraged by the openness of President Museveni, but had few government resources and international networks to draw upon. They were angry, but not at their government – which had just come to power and brought them peace and some hope for the future. Noerine Kaleeba says that her activism was driven by anger at the discrimination and stigma experienced by her husband, and by the world's double standards. She enjoins people living with HIV/AIDS (PLWHA) and their families, 'Don't despair and don't lose your anger either. I know that one day we will overcome.'[22] Another Ugandan activist, Milly Katana, says, 'We are angry. Our people are dying. We can no longer accept millions of needless AIDS deaths simply because we are poor Africans.'[23]

In South Africa, Zackie Achmat has used the 'genocide' image to describe the numbers of poor people needlessly dying. Edwin

Cameron also drew a parallel between AIDS denialists in government and the genocide denialism of some revisionist historians. His point was to compare how the two handled demonstrated facts, not to accuse the ANC of mass murder – but his carefully argued paper was misinterpreted, perhaps maliciously so.[24] The parallel between the mass murder of Jews or Rwandese and mass death from AIDS is at best inexact, but it tells us something about the political tactics of activists.

Kramer had a clear target for his anger: his government. Kaleeba, Katana and Achmat are at once more precise and more general. They are enraged by specific manifestations of stigma, denial and discrimination in the treatment of people living with HIV and AIDS. Achmat, who has most reason to be outraged at his government, selects his targets carefully: specific policies. They are also angry about a world order that gives so little value to African lives. The most powerful institutions of global governance are physically remote from Africa, but in important ways they have proved to be accessible to African activists. Outside South Africa, national governments, the classic focus for human rights critique and activist rage, have somehow been spared.

How did this happen? The answer has the following parts. It begins with the synergy between human rights activism and public health in the response to AIDS, beginning in America and developing in Africa. In parallel there has been a transformation of humanitarian action and human rights practice, driven in part by changes in Africa's position vis-à-vis the West since the end of the Cold War. Finally, and most unexpectedly, the practice of revolutionary solidarity has been taken up in America by the libertarian and religious right.

From the first days of recognizing AIDS, governments treated HIV differently from other communicable epidemic diseases. An armoury of restrictive measures exists for controlling infectious diseases, including quarantine and isolation, and mandatory testing, reporting and partner notification. Industrialized countries still have such provisions in place for some sexually transmitted infections such as syphilis (though they are rarely used in a draconian manner). They implemented similar measures in response to SARS and are ready to do so for avian flu. But from the outset AIDS was different. The American gay community was instrumental in ensuring that important guarantees on individual human rights, especially voluntary testing and strict patient confidentiality, were respected. Gay activists were afraid that their recently won gains in personal freedom might be reversed by public health controls imposed on account of AIDS, and persuasively argued that the only way to control the epidemic was with the active consent of the at-risk groups. Human rights principles were indelibly imprinted on AIDS activism. Through the work of activist civil servants, notably Jonathan Mann, democratic consent and voluntary behaviour change also became the guiding principles of the global public health response. While some Asian countries – notably Thailand – have developed national variants on the model, sub-Saharan African countries have without exception stuck faithfully to the liberal script.

Some public health specialists, among them Kevin De Cock, regret this 'AIDS exceptionalism' and argue that it is inappropriate, especially in Africa.[25] Instead, they argue for the 'normalization' of AIDS, namely 'treating HIV/AIDS more like other infectious diseases for which early diagnosis is essential for appropriate therapeutic and preventive measures, within the requirements of informed consent and respect for confidentiality'.[26] If we recognized HIV/AIDS as the emergency that it undoubtedly is, De Cock argues, we would be much more forthright in recognizing that the rights of the individual must be balanced against the well-being of the majority.

> We think that the emphasis on human rights in HIV/AIDS prevention has reduced the importance of public health and social justice, which offer a framework for prevention efforts

in Africa that might be more relevant to people's daily lives and more likely to be effective.... [O]n the basis of epidemiological data, we think that HIV/AIDS is the greatest threat to life, liberty, and the pursuit of happiness and prosperity in many African countries. Interventions, therefore, must be quantitatively and qualitatively commensurate with the magnitude of the threat posed by the disease....[27]

The ethical case is strong. The right of the non-infected to remain that way has been neglected.

But how 'exceptional' is the response to AIDS? In the third quarter of the twentieth century, the burden of responsibility for public health had shifted, from a coercive state towards a system whereby citizens bore the greater obligation for outcomes. Peter Baldwin has called this 'democratic public health' and characterized it as a system in which 'self-control, voluntary compliance, and individual responsibility rather than coercion, compulsion, and collective action were the watchwords'.[28] This has occurred mostly in Western countries, where personal liberty is linked to the discipline of good epidemiological citizenship.

Many African governments, no doubt, would have preferred to utilize the AIDS epidemic as a pretext for extending state control over the personal lives of their citizens. Where they could do this with minimal fear of a backlash – within the armed forces, for example – they have done so. Every African army that can undertake mandatory testing does it, and most of them routinely reject or dismiss individuals who test positive.[29] In the rest of society, this approach has simply been impossible. Neither, however, can African countries pursue 'democratic public health' policies and expect the same outcomes that are expected in more thickly administered, intensively health-serviced Western societies.

Baldwin's study of how industrialized countries responded to AIDS demonstrates remarkable continuities in public health practices from previous epidemics as far back as the nineteenth century.[30] In Africa, such continuity is unthinkable. Colonial medicine,[31] environmental conservation[32] and post-colonial relief and development efforts[33] have all served as mechanisms for extending state control into communities that have good reason to distrust all external authorities. Colonial medical 'campaigns' often resembled police operations, especially when 'sanitary' measures involved destroying crops and burning houses. Conservation efforts, including creating wildlife parks and 'protecting' hillsides from erosion and forests from exploitation, were often not only coercive but fundamentally misguided. Indigenous knowledge was swept aside, often with disastrous results.[34] The loss of autonomy that comes with state services may bring more difficulties than those services bring benefits. In South Africa in particular, the public health profession had a deplorable record of serving as handmaiden to apartheid while industries such as asbestos mining ravaged the health of the workforce.[35]

Anything that smacks of a return to control-based public health practice is certain to be obstructed across Africa. Violent resistance is unlikely. Discreet subversion and appeal to outside friends are more probable. Activists have already established strong alliances with international public health policy makers and have considerable clout in international forums. They have come a long way from grassroots mobilization and pulling the levers of local power. In research for this book, Kintu Nyago interviewed four Ugandan AIDS activists, and compiled a life history of a fifth, the late Bishop Misaeri Kauma. They demonstrate how Ugandan AIDS activism has been transformed in just a few years and has become an internationally networked affair.

The Right Reverend Misaeri Kauma, bishop of Namirembe Diocese, was one of the first public figures in Uganda to speak openly about AIDS in the 1980s. Alarmed by the numbers of his parishioners who were falling sick and dying, he preached openness. At first he associated AIDS with promiscuity and was resolutely opposed to condoms, but later revised his stand and is reported to have said: 'If you are foolish enough to have sinful sex, don't be so stupid not to use a condom.' The Bishop was a counsellor to people living with HIV and AIDS, an advocate for abstinence and faithfulness, and a provider of assistance to orphans. At that time, international activism on AIDS in Africa was weak to non-existent, and Ugandan activism was an entirely home-grown affair. The Bishop's ambitions were framed by local constituencies and national institutions. He became the first director-general of the government-established Ugandan AIDS Commission. In retrospect, his activist career seems oddly dated: he focused his energies entirely on his own people and saw a government post as the culmination of his activities. He was not well-connected to the NGO world, and since his death his widow Geraldine Kauma has been forced to scale back the assistance she can provide to children under her care, trying without success to gain help from international agencies and the President's wife, Janet Museveni.

The other four individuals all became active a few years later and their cases illustrate the diversity of AIDS activism and the richness of linkages between grassroots mobilization, NGO service provision, and international funding and advocacy. One example is Beatrice Were, formerly coordinator of the Community of Women Living with HIV and AIDS and subsequently AIDS coordinator for ActionAid Uganda. A social worker diagnosed HIV-positive, Beatrice focused her concern on what would happen to her children, and succeeded in mobilizing an impressive grassroots movement and attracting international support. Another example is Canon Gideon Byamugisha, an unusual instance of a pastor who has publicly declared his HIV-positive status. Chairperson of the Africa Network of Religious Leaders Living with or Personally Affected by HIV/AIDS (ANERELA), he is also an International Church Partnership Adviser for the international NGO World Vision and a resource person for UNAIDS and the World Bank. A third case is Major Rubaramira Ruranga, who has become well-known as an outspoken retired soldier. He was diagnosed with HIV in

1989 but it was participation at an international conference in the Netherlands in 1992 that gave him the confidence to think positively about his future and speak publicly about his status. Attending another conference in Mexico was the spark that encouraged him to establish an NGO, the National Guidance and Empowerment Network of People Living with HIV/AIDS (NGEN+). A final case is Dr Margaret Mungerera, a medical doctor and treatment activist, herself living with HIV. One of her innovations has been to co-found 'Mama's Club', which provides psycho-social support to HIV-positive mothers and children. She has an international profile and is a member of several African networks, including the African Treatment Preparedness Group and its international counterpart.

It is from such diverse sources with varied networks and link-ages that the response to HIV/AIDS has been patched together. It is an NGO model of response, uneven in coverage and quality, responsive to the particularities of local circumstance, the character of local leaders, and the availability and types of funds available. Given the precipitous speed with which this network has been put together, it has grown remarkably strong roots locally and internationally. It is a humane and pluralist system, concerned with civility in governance, gender equality and human rights. But, despite the fall in HIV prevalence in Uganda during the 1990s, the efficiency of this NGO model at producing epidemiological outcomes is unproven. There are many possible explanations for the Ugandan 'success story', some of which will be analysed in Chapter 5. Moreover, there are good reasons – such as those rehearsed by De Cock – for suspecting that the NGO system serves as a marketplace in which the interests of the most vocal may be met to the neglect of wider public goods. Those who dream of a 'normalized' state-based public health response to AIDS must contend not only with the vested interests in the existing patchwork, but also with the strengths of such a decentralized and adaptive system.

Transformations in Governance

The key obstacle to any control-based public health response to AIDS is that few if any African states have the capacity and legitimacy to implement a 'normal' public health response to HIV/AIDS of the scale and intrusiveness required. The AIDS pandemic has coincided with far-reaching restructuring of public service provision in Africa, with health and emergency relief in the vanguard, resulting in hybrid forms of public health organization, with a high degree of participation by national and international NGOs and foreign donors. Similar restructuring is evident in areas as diverse as journalism training and security sector reform. Twenty years ago, most African governments had a formal commitment to state-provided health, education and welfare services. In reality, most of these services were at a standstill, even before austerity measures were introduced in the vain hope that 'structural adjustment' would deliver economic growth and hence better welfare. More recently, international policy makers have rediscovered the importance of the state – though not yet one of its key roles in Western countries, the provision of universal social welfare. But the early 21st-century 'capable state' is very different to its predecessor, less from deliberate design than from the far-reaching changes in Africa's position in the world that have taken place in the meantime.

In Africa today, the formulaic ideal of democracy, in which the government presents itself and its policies to electors for approval or change, is not the main mechanism of accountability. Accountability is diffused through different mechanisms, of which the ballot box is only one. African governments are influenced by organized constituencies (increasingly 'civil society organizations' or CSOs), domestic power brokers with big constituencies or wealth, their peers (other African leaders), and international donors, creditors and investors. The most visible element in this web of relations is answerability to international donors. Critics on the left contend that external dependency weakens domestic accountability – the 'democratization of disempowerment' as the late Claude Aké described it.[36] Aké argued that the spread of formal democracy in the early 1990s came along with a wholesale transfer of sovereignty over economic and social policy to the IMF, World Bank and other Western donors. He describes the 'trivialization' of democracy: 'Democracy has been displaced by something else which has assumed its name while largely dispensing with its content.'[37]

In reality, the process is more complicated and less discouraging. During the Cold War, power was constrained within a tight ambit of domestic power brokers and external patrons. Removed from any meaningful engagement with citizens, rulers sought legitimacy through patrimony, kinship and the appropriation of spiritual authority. The Cold War thaw brought a rising tide: a series of waves that swept in and receded, slowly and unevenly bringing new political waterlines.

The 'waves' included formal democratization through multi-party elections, economic liberalization, signing on to human rights instruments, allowing national CSOs to participate in forming public policy (for example through involvement in drafting Poverty Reduction Strategy Papers, PRSPs), the adoption of a series of pan-African norms such as the unacceptability of military coups and non-constitutional transfers in power, and the creation of the African Peer Review Mechanism (APRM) for assessing political and economic governance. Each of these, taken individually, could be sceptically dismissed as a sham. In most cases, there is room for cynicism, as rhetoric flies far ahead of reality. Multi-party elections have often returned former single-party leaders or military men (but not always). Human rights conventions have been honoured in the breach as much as the observance (but there has been progress – there are far more local radios and newspapers than ever before). 'Participatory' PRSPs have often been a sham, with the recommendations written in advance by teams from the national finance ministry and the World Bank (but the second round of PRSPs was appreciably better than the first). The African Union's ban on coups was not enforced in Congo-Brazzaville and was compromised in Togo (but it was enforced in Sierra Leone, and the principle, developed to include any non-constitutional transfer of power, helped compel Zambia's Frederic Chiluba to step down). Zimbabwe is an embarrassment on many fronts. Doubtless, the first efforts of the APRM will disappoint – but the second may be better.

It is easy to sneer at norms adopted by less-than-democratic leaders and at the readiness of African presidents to sign up to international covenants that they appear to have little intention of respecting. But normative pressures work. This is because of the intersection of demanding and articulate African constituencies and the financial clout of international donors.

Non-governmental organizations are proliferating across Africa and becoming important social and political actors. The philanthropic NGO has long been decried by the left as a means of addressing only the symptoms of poverty and thus obscuring the political strategies needed to overcome it. NGOs are criticized for creating Potemkin villages not replicable at scale. Their limits are often painfully apparent. Some are 'briefcase' NGOs, to give their founders income or profile. The CSO language of 'empowerment', 'participation' and gender equality is often hot air. Questions of representation and accountability are pertinent. It is easy to be irritated by the way in which a donor-funded NGO sector has become constitutive of 'civil society'. 'Donorism' – overriding sensitivity to the concerns of funders – afflicts many CSOs. Theorists such as Mbembe rightly decry the use of 'civil society' in the African context, since African modes of power blur the distinction between state and society,[38] and government and NGO are mutually permeable entities. Individuals can move between the two: opposition leaders find the label 'NGO' convenient and the wives of government leaders set up well-protected 'NGOs'.

The NGO-CSO revolution may not match the claims of its headlines. But it has opened up new opportunities for citizens – at least those who are educated and connected to the outside world. The meaning of the term 'civil society' has itself shifted in a revealing way. Rather than an abstraction encompassing all the organized forces in society distinct from the state and those seeking political office, it now refers to those specific non-governmental organizations that donors can fund. The newly minted term 'civil societies' in the plural reflects this new operational definition. There is a sad history of funders determining the agenda of CSOs, its low point marked by the CIA funding of cultural organizations and journals in the 1950s and 1960s.[39] Donor interests, ideologies and modes of operation in Africa today are somewhat different and less malign, but they are pervasive nonetheless.

During the Cold War, the superpowers' search for clients meant that political and strategic interests triumphed. This gave client governments some room for political manoeuvre – they could threaten to defect to the opposing camp. In Washington DC, the State Department's need to reward political loyalty could trump Treasury's demands for financial accountability. In the 1980s, the competition was fierce over US policy towards countries such as Zaïre and Somalia. At the end of the decade, political alignment mattered much less. The economists' triumph was symbolized by James Baker's transfer from Treasury to State in 1989 and his immediate clampdown on the worst economic offender, Sudan. African governments became clients in search of patrons. There was no choice but to submit to the US and the Europeans and their policy frameworks – a reality illustrated by Sudan, among others, which sought funds from militant Islamist movements and was otherwise ostracized, and those, such as Liberia, which opted for criminal networks.

At first, the new frameworks were simplistic: liberal economic policies and multi-party electoral democracy. This was Aké's dependency with a liberal face. But over the 1990s, the demands became hugely more complicated, at the same time as donor governments became more transparent and the World Bank began to consult with influential NGOs. Transnational corporations became more sensitive to charges of complicity in human rights abuses, corruption or environmental despoliation. A new aid and international policy apparatus emerged, powerful but permeable. African governments could use these new channels of influence if they were light-footed – and some of them brought in CSO activists and professors to help them do that. But the real beneficiaries were African NGO leaders and African staff in international NGOs, who found they could exercise immense influence indirectly, by using foreign intermediaries to put pressure on their host governments. Margaret Keck and Kathryn Sikkink have called this the 'boomerang' pattern.[40] Blocked from direct routes of access, African activists meet with their Western counterparts, who have access to policy makers in Washington and Brussels, who in turn squeeze African governments. A fine example is the complex institutional arrangements, welfare programmes, environmental and human rights guarantees, and financial instruments surrounding the Chad–Cameroon oil pipeline. Religious constituencies are particularly significant in this emergent matrix of influence. Churches combine domestic constituencies, symbolic power and international connections. For all its shortcomings, the international NGO-CSO network has enabled African citizens to gain influence and protection.

Those shortcomings are considerable. The Chad–Cameroon pipeline also illustrates the limits of circuitous participation: the accountability mechanisms failed because the Chadian government was determined to subvert them, and the interests in civil society and human rights were too diffused and ill-organized to prevail. In most cases, participation and accountability have been limited to élites with access to education and international networks: African participation in international aid institutions can be seen as co-option rather than empowerment. In some cases, CSOs have become a distraction from the task of building representative democracy. In a parallel way, the welfare provision delivered by these NGO mechanisms is an uneven panoply of projects, neglecting basic social welfare mechanisms such as pensions and child support and disability grants. Following the mantra of avoiding dependency, the weakest and inevitably dependent members of society have been left without a safety net at all. Such political-economic systems allow for levels of extreme poverty that would have caused political crisis in any industrialized country and most middle-income countries too.[41]

African states are suspended within intangible matrices of legitimacy. Reputations matter. This is most clearly the case with the new architecture of African governance, symbolized by the African Union and the African Peer Review Mechanism. While the formal APRM itself may be languishing, an informal system of peer control is flourishing, through the norms of constitutionalism and respectability established by the African Union. African heads of state have an incentive to enforce the norms because all suffer when one lapses.

African governments are therefore located in complicated new webs of accountability, reaching downwards to new domestic players (CSOs and citizens in international agencies), sideways to other African governments, the African Union and subregional organizations, and upwards to a changed and permeable set of foreign institutions. Democratic purists fear that the face-to-face confrontation between elector and representative is becoming devalued or even lost in this profusion of channels for influence. That is indeed true, but traditional electoral encounters are declining in importance across the world, as more and more policies are decided in fora that are inaccessible to voter and parliamentarian. Arguably, Africa is negotiating a form of participation that is suitable to a continent dependent on external finance, with weak institutions and constant risk of political regression or conflict.

Just as experienced African smallholders diversify their sources of income and build up webs of assets and claims, African citizen activists are diversifying their channels of influence so as not to rely exclusively on domestic institutions and processes that are fragile and easily manipulated. The aid encounter, formerly the source of popular disenfranchisement, is becoming a source of citizens' influence and protection.

External dependency may be undesirable in general, but if it exists it is better for dependents to be able to get the best out of the system. As political power becomes distributed in a permeable transnational system of national and foreign governments, multilateral organizations and international NGOs, it makes sense for African citizens to find mechanisms for accessing those networks to secure protection, funds and influence. And they are doing so with some success, bringing benefits to those who participate and their constituencies. This helps stabilize an increasingly civil and rights-oriented governance system that is a distinct improvement on the past. But this involves a consensual charade. Donor and recipient publicly claim that the purpose of their partnership is to deliver services such as reducing poverty or overcoming HIV/AIDS. Sometimes this happens. The more consistent outcome is that donors obtain the cooperation of local actors in their intrusion into Africa, while the local actors become more secure.

Such a system can be played from all sides. Activists may be able to manage a bad leader by circumventing and reducing his power, without having to resort to the old all-or-nothing strategy of outright confrontation. But it also means that a skilful ruler can appease a range of stakeholders to stay in office, and reward the old-style power brokers such as the army. Uganda's President Yoweri Museveni has been particularly adept at this. We should also be clear that African constituencies and concerns do not actually drive this machine. African subalterns are deftly exploiting opportunities in a global framework.

Nowhere are these transformations, with all their opportunities and problems, more apparent than with HIV/AIDS. The emergent AIDS apparatus is an exaggerated version of the existing aid and policy mechanisms with some peculiar features of its own. It includes host governments, local CSOs, AIDS activists and organizations of people living with HIV and AIDS, international NGOs, private foundations, governmental donors, multilateral institutions, special new funding mechanisms, global advocacy networks, pharmaceutical companies, militaries, contractors, scientists, religious zealots, and a host of others. Because the apparatus of international AIDS governance is new and flexible it has attracted a range of groups and agendas that seek legitimacy and progress through association. Because it has so much money it is attracting real power brokers.

Perhaps the most astonishing aspect of African AIDS activism has been its success in attracting resources and representing AIDS constituencies. People living with HIV and AIDS are among the most marginalized people in the most powerless continent, but a string of successes have been scored by them or on their behalf. One success is making it legally unacceptable to discriminate against people living with HIV and AIDS. *De facto* discrimination is widespread, but whenever it is challenged the law is clear. Another victory was establishing the Global Fund to fight AIDS, TB and Malaria in 2001, alongside a huge increase in funding for AIDS through existing mechanisms. Donor resources for AIDS in Africa have risen tenfold between 1996 and 2005, and most of this is new money. Perhaps most dramatic was the precipitous fall in the price of antiretroviral drugs between 2001 and 2003, so that they became an affordable option in poor countries. From the point of view of the activists and their supporters these victories are only right and natural, because of the scale of the problem they are facing and the objective needs for resources this entails. Compared with the other deserving causes, the successes are remarkable. The immediate impact has been to put AIDS ineradicably on the agenda. In the longer term, it holds the promise of truly grappling with the epidemic.

A considerable number of these activists have joined international organizations such as NGOs and multilateral agencies, finding allies there. Milly Katana serves on the board of the Global Fund. Unlike militants of earlier generations who waged their struggles clandestinely from within hostile institutions, these AIDS activists have been embraced by the international agencies precisely because of their outspokenness. They may not have stormed the domestic citadel but they have been invited into the remoter halls of power where the financing of those citadels is determined, and they have become part of the new globalized network of African governance.

New Solidarities

The transformations in African governance of the last two decades have gone hand-in-hand with commensurate changes in the nature of humanitarian action and human rights practice, and the relationship of activists to state power. This has taken different paths in the US and in Europe.

Any militant movement is defined by its adversaries. In the case of the first American AIDS activists these adversaries included the Reagan administration, the medical establishment, and conservative Christians. A rapprochement with the pharmaceutical companies and scientists was not long in coming, as gay men became highly literate in medical science and enthusiastic participants in drug trials. An accommodation with the Republican Party and the Christian Right seemed out of the question. This has now happened, albeit in the somewhat removed and neutral space that Africa occupies in US politics. The President's Emergency Program for AIDS Relief (PEPFAR) is the world's largest AIDS donor. This could be seen as another accident of history, born of the opportunism of circumstance, as George W. Bush sought a charitable dimension to his administration's foreign policy, and another zig-zag in AIDS's bizarre trajectory across the political spectrum.

On closer inspection, the coming-together of AIDS, humanitarianism, human rights, and a Republican foreign policy is less unexpected. Humanitarian action burst out of its Cold War straitjacket in the early 1990s, engaging in a host of new situations (especially civil wars), expanding mandates to deal with human rights and conflict resolution as well as traditionally charitable activities, and at times calling for international military action in pursuit of security or an end to human rights violations. The 'humanitarian international' has long had an ambiguous regard for international law. While international agencies recognize that their activities are almost always made possible and safe by multilateral norms and international humanitarian law, they also have a record of overriding legality when they think it is immoral – providing aid to civilians in secessionist Biafra, or citizens of embargoed Cambodia, for example. Humanitarian action is ultimately concerned with outcomes, and if a remedy can be snatched beyond the reach of law, the more assertive humanitarians have no qualms in calling for military intervention or regime change. A similar progression is made by some liberals and human rights advocates, who call for decisive action to remove oppressive governments. If national sovereignty clashes with fundamental human rights, they argue, human rights should win. The logic is that solidarity with the oppressed dictates using force to liberate them, and if that force is available, it should be used. Thus, liberal social democrats in government – such as Tony Blair – find sound moral arguments for supporting forcible regime change in Iraq, even though it is evident that America's intervention is driven by completely different priorities. The intervention in Iraq confounds the categories left and right: many on the left who criticize it do so either from visceral dislike of President Bush or from attachment to a rather conservative set of multilateral principles. It is the Bush administration, using power for ideological ends as well as self-interest, which is revolutionary, or at least Napoleonic.

The polarization of American political discourse, especially over foreign policy, conceals some common threads that unite diverse constituencies. The strongest of these is a salvation agenda, a belief that a combination of money, technology and goodwill can solve any problem. Religious communities add 'faith' as well. In the eye of the donating public, humanitarians act according to a script in which they bring some kind of salvation to unfortunate victims. It is largely a fantasy, but it provides a popular underpinning for both military liberation and foreign aid. The salvation narrative has roots in Christian charity and resonance with an American exceptionalist view of the rest of the world.[42]

Even histories of the AIDS epidemic succumb to the salvation narrative structure. Randy Shilts's *And the Band Played On*[43] ranks as a semi-official account of the early years of AIDS in America, in which American gay activists, alongside physicians, epidemiologists and some public health officers, play the role of narrative heroes. Unfortunately there is no redemption in sight, and the heroes are ultimately tragic. As the story shifts from American city hospitals to central Africa, Haiti and India, the doctor and public health worker also take on the mantle of adventurer and missionary, braving the perils of war, superstition and primitive sanitary conditions in a tropical jungle. The finest exponents of this genre include Laurie Garrett[44] and Greg Behrman.[45] The power of science, unshackled from bureaucratic impediment and popular ignorance and fear, can conquer our enemies. The supporting cast includes advocate economists such as Jeffrey Sachs – who argues that the money is available and is an insignificant part of Western budgets – and rock stars such as Bono. Africa is partly scenery, and Africans are mostly extras, save occasional sub-heroes such as Museveni and (too rarely) Noerine Kaleeba or Philly Lutaaya.

Secular humanitarians, interventionist liberals and Christian missionaries all share a faith in the transformative potential of American power. Theirs is an unfinished script that anticipates a heroic denouement.

In this light, Bush's embrace of HIV/AIDS is quite consistent. The logic of the salvation agenda is that Americans can exercise practical solidarity with oppressed and poor people across the world, offering them real (if American) solutions to their predicaments. These solutions are selective and come with many strings attached, including an unambiguous moral agenda that limits funds to family planning providers (the global gag rule) and to prevention efforts that promote condom use. Consonant with the individualizing impetus of 'democratic public health', the message is always to stress individual responsibility. The libertarian-Christian coalition has created a new solidarity, which has a power centre on the right but which has adopted some of the left's ideals, including liberty and solidarity with those who are suffering. This new solidarity takes seriously America's mission of saving the rest of the world from itself. The US has changed from being a *status quo* power to promoting revolutionary transformation, albeit selectively. This may be a brief period before service as normal resumes, but at the minimum it will leave its imprint on America and the world for a long time to come.

Meanwhile, a different strand of internationalism is dominant in Europe, driven by rights and cooperation rather than by solidarity and salvation (with Tony Blair perhaps representing the meeting point of the different strands). This approach to international welfare emphasizes the importance of the state and social democratic social contracts. The European model has also emphasized NGOs and neglected social welfare entitlements, but as the experiment in taking aid resources to scale is pursued, it may well fall back upon universal child benefit or old age pension schemes as a mechanism for poverty reduction in Africa. Just as the TAC has encouraged South African social activists to campaign for a basic income grant and judicially enforceable social and economic rights, the successes of international AIDS activism may inspire new, entitlement-based models of aid-driven poverty reduction.

Africa's AIDS activists have not needed to stage revolutions at home. They have been part of an international revolution and have entered welcoming citadels far more powerful than any they could have dreamed of storming. Their interests are better represented than ever before, their rights better protected. AIDS activism has certainly helped secure liberal governance and has obtained vast funds for its agenda. For many activists their struggle is a race against time. Those who are living with HIV and AIDS are acutely aware of their reliance on drugs with probable side-effects and a time horizon of efficacy. Many are also fearful that AIDS's long wave of illness and death could overwhelm their fragile societies.

4

How African Democracies
Withstand AIDS

The Issue of a Lifetime

Could AIDS so damage the socio-political fabric as to cause social chaos and political upheaval? Could all the brave work of AIDS activists and policy makers to mobilize funds and support human rights and participation be swamped by social calamity? So far, this has not occurred. Although the worst of the epidemic is yet to come, and judging the likely impacts of HIV/AIDS on society is remarkably difficult, the evidence to date suggests that African social and political systems will absorb the impact of HIV/AIDS, albeit at a very high cost, borne chiefly by poor women.

This chapter deals with conjectures about what might happen – in most cases explaining why fears are real, but easily exaggerated. The discussion rests on an analytical framework for examining various ways in which endemic AIDS could threaten democracy. The chapter criticizes the evidence and theory of this framework (which, in the spirit of self-critical dialectic, is chosen from my own writings).

The analytical framework relates adult life expectancy to complex institutions and modern governance, creating a multidimensional process model for the impact of endemic HIV/AIDS on society.[1] The hypothesis is that a major and prolonged drop in adult life expectancy will make it difficult to sustain modern institutions. Most projections for what AIDS might do to societies are extraordinarily simplistic, little more than a catalogue of potential disasters without any connecting theoretical thread. The relationship between life expectancy and social complexity provides such a connecting thread. The driver of change in the model is not AIDS itself but life expectancy. Alongside the data for HIV prevalence – figures that in themselves have no obvious socio-political import – the one overriding and truly empirical measure of distress in a society is life expectancy. But the implications of a major and sustained drop in adult life expectancy have gone largely unremarked. Across southern Africa, life expectancy began to plummet in the 1990s and is expected to continue falling until at least 2010.

As noted in the opening pages of this book, the normal measure used – life expectancy at birth – understates the gravity of what is occurring in Africa today, because adults are dying of AIDS. Additional life expectancy on attaining adulthood (say at age fifteen or twenty) is a better indicator of the subjective expectation of longevity and a better measure of how the life expectancy changes might impact upon life decisions and economic rationality.

Compare South Africa and Chad in 2000. Both had life expectancies at birth of fifty years. But Chad followed a more traditional African pattern, with half of the deaths being children under five. Having survived the hazards of childhood, a Chadian teenager could expect to live to over sixty, approximately a 'normal' adult life of four or five decades. She or he could expect to bear children and grandchildren, and pursue a career through to retirement. South Africa was following a different, AIDS-impacted demographic pattern. Just 15 per cent of deaths were of young children. More than half of South African teenagers could expect to die before they reached sixty. And South Africa was just beginning to feel the impact of AIDS mortality. By 2005, Chadian adult life expectancy was five years longer than South African. As this march of death continued, most young South Africans could no longer expect to live to see their children into maturity and greet their grandchildren; most would never pursue a career until retirement, or be able to take out a 25-year mortgage to buy a house.

A crucial hinge of this argument is how objective measures of longevity translate into subjective expectations of life. This is a field that needs social-psychological and anthropological inquiry. One can hypothesize that anticipated longevity is a function of cultural and religious norms, individual outlook, and life experience – including observing the ages of death of one's elders and one's peers. With a slow-moving endemic, the cultural and perceptual shifts might take a generation or more to occur, lagging well behind the curve of AIDS deaths.

How could it *not* be the case that this calamitous fall in adult life expectancy would *not* have far-reaching impacts on society? It will create the most marked divergence in global life chances for a century – and possibly sustain this global inequity indefinitely. Surely, over time, the expectation of dying in what we call 'mid-life' should change rational behaviour, creating a new *Homo economicus* and *Homo politicus*? Moreover, the changes would be systemic across society, and would represent changes in trajectories of change. The basic idea for what might happen to societies is borrowed and adapted from Malcolm McPherson, who argued that, just as economic development was best seen as a process, the impact of massive loss of human capital should also be seen as a process. 'Running Adam Smith in reverse' was his telling phrase.[2] Instead of a gradual accumulation of capital, with human capital increases spilling over into greater investment in physical capital, an economy that was losing adults would begin to suffer from an erosion of all kinds of capital. The model develops this hypothesis in three main areas: institutional and political development, the demographic transition, and – following McPherson – economic growth.

'Weber in Reverse'

In the same idiom as McPherson's 'Adam Smith in reverse', institutional development, hypothetically, could follow the trajectory of 'Max Weber in reverse'. The basic idea is illustrated by a comparison between a sophisticated bureaucracy run on rational principles – say a university administration – and an organization that relies on charisma and immediate interest to mobilize – say a student union. In the provost's office, there will be people who have built careers over decades, with a depth of experience and a network of contacts that surpass their formidable formal qualifications. Anticipating careers of the same length and slow ascent, their underlings will studiously accumulate the same set of advantages – experience, networks and qualifications -- investing their time in the expectation of a slow return decades hence. Across the street, by contrast, the president and other officers of the student union are in post for just a year. With little experience, narrower networks and no administrative qualifications, they will cajole, promise, bully and charm their constituents, and rarely win their encounters with the clever and patient bureaucrats they confront.

The implication was that, as AIDS deaths forced a complex institution such as a government ministry or army brigade to employ people with less experience and shorter career prospects, the organizational model would shift from the 'university administration' model towards the 'student union' one. Lacking the middle managers and sergeant-majors who keep a complicated organization functioning, these institutions would become more paralytic and inefficient, but perhaps be intermittently galvanized into action by charismatic appeal, bribery or threat. The metaphor of 'hollowing out' of institutions by AIDS illness and death fails to do justice to this different – and regressive – way of doing business.

Applied to a whole government, the implication was that countries with low life expectancy would find it difficult to sustain the complicated, rule-bound systems necessary for modern democracy. Their institutions would slowly grind to a halt. In contrast to the familiar symptoms of state failure – violent conflict and civil disorder – we would see a much quieter form of paralysis. States might end with a whimper rather than a bang. Meanwhile, the pattern of political governance would regress to more traditional, authoritarian structures and even to personal rule. AIDS would create new patterns of power – or recreate old ones.

Such regression could have both institutional and cultural dimensions.[3] The specific formal and informal organizations needed for democracy to function might fail – indeed, might be among the first to do so. Those institutions include: electoral commissions and related organizations, parliaments and local councils, and political parties. How might these be affected by AIDS? Several researchers – including Bob Mattes,[4] Per Strand[5] and Samantha Willan[6] – have investigated these issues, looking at South Africa. They see real but not disastrous impacts, but warn that this may change in the future as the epidemic matures. Burdens imposed by AIDS include more frequent by-elections, extra effort to keep the electoral roll up-to-date, loss of skills and efficiency in electoral institutions, and making provision for the sick and infirm to cast their votes.

In South Africa, the number of by-elections has increased since about 2000, putting additional financial and administrative demands on the electoral system. Running elections demands a skilled workforce with an institutional memory (particularly important given that there is usually a five-year gap between elections). South Africa relies on a core of trained personnel, plus a large number of volunteers and enlisted short-term staff, many of them teachers. All of these occupational groups suffer high rates of HIV, although turnover has been reduced by anti-retroviral treatment. These problems are common to complex institutions in AIDS-affected countries, but have particular significance where such important events as elections are involved.

Fair and credible elections depend upon an up-to-date electoral roll. As AIDS deaths increase, the removal of dead voters from the voters roll becomes an increasingly demanding function, complicated by under-registration of deaths. Africa is plagued with allegations of foul play around issues of 'ghost voters' at the best of times, and such high death rates may well heighten suspicion and rejection of election outcomes.

Rising levels of illness in the country place increased demands on the electoral system to provide additional special ways of voting for the infirm, and more voting stations so that the sick are not expected to travel long distances. For the 2004 election, South Africa's Independent Electoral Commission (IEC) required all municipal electoral officers to visit all citizens who were in hospital or bed-ridden to register them for voting, and to visit them again during the election so that they could cast their votes.[7] This is commendable but costly. Voter registration also becomes more complicated as both voters and IEC staff become sick, over-burdened or disillusioned.

In research commissioned for this book, Ephraim Kimotho interviewed Kenyan MPs, councillors, parliamentary staff and members of the Electoral Commission of Kenya (ECK). One of the most striking findings was the time and financial burdens on elected representatives arising from the increased hardships and more frequent deaths of constituents. MPs and councillors are expected to organize and participate in a range of fundraising activities, with local cooperatives and 'Harambee' events. In the past, these activities were mostly for community development. Today, 85 per cent of those interviewed estimated that most of their fundraising was for constituents' medical bills. They estimated that 30 per cent of their time is spent in churches, attending funerals and fundraising events. This bears out a remark by Justin Malewezi, a Malawian MP and former vice-president, who said that 'a member of parliament sees the face of AIDS almost every day'.[8]

Political authority in Kenya is often organized around powerful local families, which become champions of their localities, but by the same token hold the fortunes of that area in their hands. One councillor in Machakos told Kimotho: 'This is the problem in our country. The churches, cooperative societies, political parties and community programmes are all run by members of the same families. If they die, they die with our dreams and programmes. If they fall victim of HIV/AIDS they use our resources to support themselves.' The loss of even one powerful individual can bring poverty or political crisis on an entire council, or indeed a government. High-ranking party members interviewed by Kimotho recognized the vulnerability of the political leadership, but it was notable that AIDS was pushed into the political background by the campaign over the new national constitution.

In Kenya as elsewhere, the pace of by-elections due to incumbent deaths has picked up. Eighteen MPs died in office over the ten years between July 1993 and July 2003, eleven of them since 1998. These by-elections are expensive. But a decrease in the number of vacant seats due to electoral petitions and defections has meant that the overall number of by-elections has not increased. It is estimated that between four and five parliamentary staff die each year from HIV/AIDS and related illnesses.

Kimotho's research identified two possible distortions of the democratic process itself. One is the existence of large numbers of 'ghost voters' who have died but have not been removed from the electoral roll. A 2002 study by the IEC estimated that 15.8 per cent of registered voters were in fact dead. Anecdotal reports from subsequent elections indicate that some of these individuals appear to have cast votes, and in some constituencies the voter turnout exceeded the living electors. The problem of electoral fraud is compounded by even larger problems with voter registration: it can take as many as nine trips to the central office in Nairobi to collect an ID card. There are an estimated 1.4 million uncollected voter identity cards nationwide, nearly half in Nairobi alone. Unlike South Africa, Kenya has no special provisions for the infirm or incapacitated to be helped to vote. These factors together make it easier for votes to be rigged.

A second problem is vote buying, especially among poor female voters, many of whom have to pay medical bills or support orphaned children. Sixty per cent of the MPs and councillors said that they focus their campaign efforts on women, and one young woman in Naivasha commented: 'I cannot go hungry if I sell my vote.' Vote buying is most efficiently done at party primaries, where turnout is low.

Other institutions that might fade or fail include police forces, the judiciary and local government. The inefficiency, paralysis or collapse of any of these spells trouble. A rare study on local government was carried out by Ryann Manning on how the epidemic was affecting the eThekweni Municipality in KwaZulu-Natal. Manning set out to examine whether HIV/AIDS will undermine the capacity of local-level democratic institutions to govern effectively, reduce the capacity of municipal departments to provide public services, and increase the demand for services.[9] Her key finding was that, as early as 2002, the municipality was noticing an impact. It varied across departments, depending on a range of factors. For instance, the cemeteries department faced an increased workload, but found it relatively straightforward to plan for expanding demand. Gravediggers are unskilled and new ones can easily be recruited. By contrast, the housing department faced a more complicated situation. AIDS was depleting its skilled and experienced workforce, and it was finding it very difficult to plan strategically for housing needs in the future. Increasing numbers of orphans and changing family structures made for unpredictable changes. The fire department reported that AIDS was having a significant impact, because it was undermining the fitness of a workforce that needed to be in excellent health. In addition, fire department managers were concerned that, although they could give initial training to replacement fire-fighters in three months, it would take years for new staff to gain the necessary experience.[10]

The elected council of eThekweni was also directly hit by AIDS. Manning analysed data on councillors' reasons for missing meetings and concluded that 'if the trends are accurate, they show that a growing proportion of councillor absences are the result of illness, and that the absolute number of ill-health absences is growing'.[11]

Democracy requires political parties. In principle, the loss of key cadres could make disciplined and thoughtful parties into institutions that are more like gangs, poorly run and motivated by greed and fear. Kenyan party leaders are worried about this. Data from South Africa do not show this, at least for now. However, Willan does find evidence that parties in areas of high HIV prevalence are feeling the impact. The Inkatha Freedom Party is based in KwaZulu-Natal, the province with the highest HIV prevalence. Members responded to questions by Per Strand and his colleagues about 'impact on party', noting that they were already experiencing a strain, with members, staff and leaders falling ill and dying.[12] While HIV/AIDS may erode their support base, it may also be a push factor leading the party to address the epidemic more comprehensively. Manning found that community organizations in KwaZulu-Natal were under severe stress from AIDS. Not only were they losing staff to sickness and death, but they were under pressure to focus their activities on AIDS-related activities, to the neglect of civic education and similar activities in the political realm.

There is some speculation that HIV/AIDS might weaken the cultural preconditions for democracy. Democracies require citizens who believe in the rule of law, who are committed to core values of tolerance and pluralism, who are engaged in the civic life of their nations – and who are ready and able to turn out and vote. Could these conditions be more difficult to meet in future? Could people become exhausted and withdraw from public life, or turn their attention to caring for the sick and orphans?

Per Strand and his colleagues examined voter turnout in the 2004 election in South Africa. They found some evidence for voters being exhausted or unable to participate, either because of sickness or because of caring for the sick. Turnout was down on the previous two elections at just 57.5 per cent of the electorate. But it seems probable that the main explanation for this was that in 1994 and 1999 the very fact of voting was so historic that people turned out in enormous numbers, and a fall-off was therefore inevitable. Chapter 3 has shown that there is no consistent pattern of civil society engagement being either increased or diminished by the burdens of AIDS.

More fundamentally we might expect that a dramatic truncation of adult longevity would lead to a different rationality for decision making, a new *Homo politicus*: a change in political culture to one marked by despair, opportunism, and short time horizons. In principle this could be measured by monitoring corruption and preference for activities with quick rewards. In practice, these activities are so complicated and there are so many confounding factors that it would be remarkably difficult to establish definitive measures.

The 'Weber in reverse' model in the 2003 paper 'How Will HIV/AIDS Transform African Governance' was delightfully sophisticated and almost completely unverifiable. As Mattes and Manning noted, it is founded on logic and conjecture, rather than on empirical evidence.[13] Moreover the 'Weber in reverse' image didn't catch on. The paper was written as a challenge to the pedestrian narrative that passed for theory in most of the AIDS and governance and AIDS and security literature. Instead of sparking a theoretical debate, it is merely cited as one more reference in the rag-tag bibliographies in Africa's literature of AIDS-related doom.

A simple empirical test of the 'AIDS imperils democracy' hypothesis is the number of functioning democracies in Africa. Confounding such an expectation, this number has risen during the AIDS epidemic and continues to rise. Is this refutation or merely a challenge that requires us to refine the hypothesis?

Could it be that political retrogression is concealed by a façade of democracy? Given that any hypothesis that hinges on adult longevity requires a generation (at least) before it can be tested adequately, are we simply trying to come to judgement much too soon? Could activists' efforts to sustain democracy be doomed?

How Do African States 'Really' Function?

The model's fatal weak point is elsewhere. It contains a flawed assumption, which is that Africa's governing institutions were not only on a Weberian path, but had achieved a significant degree of rational efficiency.[14] A rich and persuasive social and political science literature demonstrates that this is not the case.[15] Social and political scientists may disagree – sometimes markedly – over the dominant characteristics of African states, but they do agree on this one point: they don't follow Western models. Governing systems may be patrimonial, wasteful and even criminal, but they 'work' – at least for those in power. They may present one face to their domestic public and another to the rest of the world, and may be adept at developing hybrid forms of political organization that combine bureaucracy and patrimonialism. And the very factors that make them surprisingly resilient in the face of permanent political and economic crisis, mean that they are well-constructed to withstand the dreadful human attrition caused by AIDS.

Most political systems are hugely wasteful of human resources and Africa is no exception. The World Bank reflected on the fact that Africa had enjoyed substantial investment in schools and universities and moaned, 'where has all the education gone?'[16] Much of Africa's expertise is abroad, and much of it internally unemployed – it is less acceptable today to keep people in prison or assassinate them, but tens of thousands of talented and qualified individuals are idle, reduced to fruitless scheming, or engaged in making a living from exploiting the opportunities for getting a private income at the expense of the general well-being. In many African countries, the political and economic incentives are so structured that it makes most sense to spend one's time and talents on individually profitable activities that do not promote social or economic development. Many clever people exploit niches such as smuggling or directing state or aid funds into personal enterprises.

Even after the depletion of AIDS, emigration of the skilled and political exile, African states still possess more trained personnel than they did at independence. States can be run – modestly – on far fewer people than are available. Some rulers continually pick out aspiring politicians – the more inexperienced the better – give them high positions, and then discard them after a couple of years. Others rely entirely on a very narrow circle of confidantes, often from their own ethnic group. Where the stress is felt is in service delivery, where health systems, schools and judiciaries are failing to deliver.

The case of militaries is a powerful illustration of the gap between model and reality. A common argument in the literature on AIDS and national security is that armies are especially at risk from HIV/AIDS. First, HIV rates among soldiers are said to be invariably much higher than in the general population. Second, this is said to lead to institutional crisis. In turn, this is said to endanger national security.[17] All three claims are questionable and are based on assumptions about military institutions and international relations that simply do not hold up. To begin with, evidence suggests that HIV rates in African armies are highly variable, usually comparable to those in civilian populations, and sometimes lower.[18] Second, a well-run professional army is designed to cope with losing personnel, and has built-in redundancy as a result. Losing men to AIDS is not intrinsically different to losing them in battle or to disease while on operations. A poorly run army tends to have even greater redundancy, encumbered with an overstaffed and over-promoted officer corps, for example. Mobutu Sese Seko had no fewer than six parallel security agencies at one point, and a national army that was so poorly equipped it was no threat to anybody, especially not − by design − to its commander-in-chief. What possible negative impact could people dying of AIDS have on such systems, already paralysed by their own leaders?

It is also instructive to note that most African armies have been rather poor at fighting guerrillas. Anyone who has tried to make a complex institution do something other than simply exist will sympathize with the plight of the general whose brigade is tied down by the logistical demands of provisioning itself and moving camp, constantly out-manoeuvred by small bands of light-footed irregulars. The student union can be a more effective form of mobilization than the provost's office. Some of the most effective programmes of social action in Africa have been undertaken in campaign mode by energetic but inexperienced political move-ments. Radical new governments often have an early and brief window of energy to implement land reform, mount literacy campaigns, and overhaul decrepit political systems. In Uganda, a young leftist guerrilla-turned-president, contemptuous of the old order, waged a campaign against AIDS in that early moment of fervour.

Africa's democratic processes must also be seen in their own light. Aziz Rana notes that 'Hopes for democracy in Africa rest on three pillars − material progress, independence from external control and the functioning of constitutional procedures.'[19] This is reflected in the first Afrobarometer survey, in which 89 per cent of southern Africans felt that access to basic provisions was an important element of democracy. The TAC has tapped into this with its stress on social and economic rights. Michael Schatzberg makes a strong case for locating democracy within a matrix of legitimacy, with axes that include the family and food. The head of state is envisioned as the 'father', both stern and caring, while a central idiom of politics is 'eating': sharing the wealth of the nation.[20]

In his study of Senegal, *Democracy in Translation*, Frederic Schaffer analyses the Wolof word *demokaraasi*, emphasizing that it refers to mechanisms for ensuring that leaders share their wealth and patronage with all members of their constituency.[21] An election is not an exercise in accountability but a means of generating communal solidarity. The TAC's strategy of building consensus rather than focusing on adversarial political competition reflects this approach, too.

The importance of sovereign independence is often overlooked by overseas policy makers. Independence is hugely prized in countries that were under colonial rule just a generation or two ago. But, as many analysts have pointed out, independence is somewhat fictional if a government is unable to make real choices over its social and economic policies.

A pessimistic reading of this evidence is that African polities can absorb many of the adverse impacts of AIDS, but only because they are already so dysfunctional at providing the basic functions of governance. By implication, the losses and stresses of HIV/AIDS are no worse than the misgovernment and war that have disfigured the continent for so long. Progress towards meeting goals for health and education will be severely shackled by shortages of skilled people, in part because of AIDS.

A more optimistic reading would emphasize that African political systems have adjusted to cope with the continent's recurrent afflictions. Modest but real progress towards peace and slow democratization will not be blown off course by the AIDS epidemic.

Democratic Demographics

The AIDS endemic is not a Malthusian crisis. Demographic predictions suggest that only in the highest-prevalence countries in southern Africa is population growth likely to be halted or perhaps slightly reversed, and that this is due in part to a trend towards lower fertility that pre-dated AIDS. Before AIDS, Africa had largely completed the first stage of the demographic transition – death rates had come down – and was entering the second phase, as birth rates began to drop. Population growth was slowing, a trend that continues with AIDS. But this apparent continuity masks important demographic changes that could have far-reaching implications for social and political stability, and hence democracy.

Applying the 'AIDS reverses processes' model to demographics, we are obliged to ask, might endemic AIDS reverse the demographic transition? This would occur through one or more of several parallel processes. First, a perceived population crisis might encourage a resurgence of pro-natalist culture, encouraging young women to marry early and have more children. Second, a decline in female education might have the same effect. Third, a shortage of adult women – as AIDS kills more women than men, and at earlier ages – might encourage men to seek out younger marriage partners. All of these are theoretically possible. There is no substantial evidence for any of them, though anecdotes lean towards the 'men taking younger partners' hypothesis.

The sex ratio imbalance among adults is a particular concern. All African populations in modern times have had a balanced sex ratio, with slightly fewer women than the pro-female populations of Western Europe, but markedly more than the male-leaning populations of China, northern India and Pakistan. The impending gender imbalance among adults in sub-Saharan Africa has no recent precedents in the continent. (The depredations of the slave trade may be an example worthy of study.) This is an area in which our knowledge is simply blank.

Another line of argument is the conjecture that AIDS would intensify a youth-skewed population imbalance. This is the 'security demographic' theory. Martin Schönteich of the Institute of Security Studies (ISS) in Pretoria first raised the alarm that South Africa's AIDS epidemic might lead to a disproportionate number of young men (a 'youth bulge') in the population that would risk increasing the crime rate, and this would be compounded by poor socialization of orphans.[22] The core of the argument is simple: most crime is committed by young men aged 15–24, and so if the proportion of that group within the population increases, crime rates are likely to rise. Prima facie, there is a case. But crime is determined by much more than demographics. More recently, Schönteich's colleagues at the ISS have reviewed the evidence and concluded that it shows that his fear was overstated.[23] A wider and more thorough review of the 'security demographic' argument, covering all continents and the period 1950–2000, concludes that there is evidence for a 'youth bulge' in the population contributing to greater risk of civil strife, especially when combined with economic stress. This is reason for general concern. Intriguingly, the review found that this association has disappeared in the post-Cold War period.[24]

A convergent strand in the literature stresses how orphaned children could be a cause of social breakdown, crime and even terrorism. With clear echoes of the 'coming anarchy' hypothesis advanced by Robert Kaplan, who considered the youth of Liberia and Sierra Leone to be 'like loose molecules in a very unstable social fluid, a fluid that was clearly on the verge of igniting',[25] it is another intuitively resonant argument. In January 2005, Trevor Nielsen of the Global Business Coalition on AIDS asserted that 'the link between AIDS, economics and terrorism is a clear and emerging threat' and singled out children orphaned by AIDS as the chief suspects.

Nielsen is not a philanthropist and he does not appeal for an end to human suffering on purely ethical grounds. As a business leader accustomed to dealing with politicians, he knows that calling on enlightened self-interest will be a better means of getting the world's business and political leaders to act on the plight of African children orphaned by AIDS. He made the following argument:[26]

Terrorist organizations establishing a foothold in Africa will find it rich for recruitment. Sub-Saharan Africa is in the midst of an orphan crisis. UNICEF estimates that 12 million children under 15 in sub-Saharan Africa have lost at least one parent to AIDS and that there will be 20 million orphans in Africa by 2010.

Although little research has been done on the link between the orphan crisis and terrorism, it is undeniable that AIDS, and the deadly conflicts that have ravaged Africa, have created a steady stream of orphans that can be exploited and used for terrorist activities.

Without caring adults to protect them, children can be manipulated into doing almost anything. Hundreds of thousands of children as young as 10 years old have been forced to fight in Angola, Ethiopia, Uganda, Sierra Leone, Rwanda, Sudan, Congo and other African countries. Amnesty International has documented that troops in the Democratic Republic of Congo routinely forced children to rape civilians and engage in cannibalism.[27] In Liberia, children have been forced to wear wigs and women's dresses in an effort to confuse opposing fighters.[28]

However, not all children are forced to become fighters. Some join out of desperation. The AIDS epidemic has created thousands of parentless households headed by children as young as five,[29] and armed groups are often the only entities that can provide children with the basic necessities to secure food, water and shelter for themselves and their siblings.

The use of children to commit terrorist acts is not new. The Islamic Jihad has been running schools to teach children how to become suicide bombers (and thus martyrs) for years.[30]

Nielson's case has no discernible empirical foundation and consists of a string of non-sequiturs, several of which have been footnoted in the summary given above. More importantly, sufficient research has been done to expose the weaknesses in the

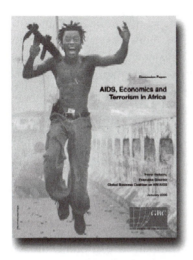

AIDS, Economics and
Terrorism in Africa

Does this represent the future for Africa's children orphaned by AIDS?

related argument, that 'orphans become delinquents'. In 2003, Rachel Bray analysed the argument and summarized existing evidence.[31] Broadly following Bray, we can break the issue down into a set of questions.

First, is the number of orphans increasing? The answer is clear: it is. This is tragedy enough and sufficient warrant for our concern. Millions of children are losing their parents and many of them are living painful and short lives themselves. AIDS particularly increases the numbers of double orphans – those who have lost both parents. It is a horrendous situation. We could add that an approach that identifies orphans as a security risk runs a risk of further stigmatizing and ostracizing those children – and possibly contributing to any emergent problems of anti-social behaviour. But while the *totals* are going up sharply, the *proportion* of Africa's children who are orphaned is rising only marginally. This is because the overall population is increasing and the numbers of children orphaned by other causes are declining. In looking at aggregates, however, we are in danger of being misled. In certain places, the burden of orphans is exceptionally severe.

Second, are these orphans overwhelming society's capacity to care for them? For the most part, it appears not. The key point here is that Africa's experience of and capacity for foster care is much wider than its experience of orphanhood. For example, a famine may not kill a significant number of adults, but it may cause mass distress migration and increased child abandonment. The drought-famine of 1984–5 in Sudan created few orphans but left hundreds of thousands of children effectively fatherless as men migrated to look for work, and thousands effectively without parental care as they were left in the care of relatives and sometimes strangers.[32] In West Africa, it is customary for children to live with foster families (usually relatives) for substantial parts of their childhood to obtain a Koranic education or formal schooling. In many societies girls are loaned to assist in the household of grandparents or relatives who have no daughter of their own. In the Sahel it is customary for boys to leave home to wander from one Sufi lodge to another, seeking an Islamic education and a patron. In southern Africa the history of labour migration and apartheid has meant that families have long been disrupted, and a large proportion of children have lived without 'normal' family life for generations.[33] The fosterage capacity of African societies is complicated and may be rather more substantial than anticipated.

Different kinds of fosterage need to be distinguished. Where it is voluntary or planned it is likely to be a much more positive experience for the child, but where it is involuntary it is less likely to be so. The AIDS crisis is probably shifting the balance between these two broad categories.

We should not be complacent and we must be alert to the places where orphan numbers and needs are truly overwhelming. In Makete district of south-west Tanzania, for example, multiple concurrent shocks – a high prevalence of HIV/AIDS being one – have led to a very severe local crisis, which includes significant numbers of orphaned children whom the community is struggling to support.[34] In hard-hit parts of western Kenya, this is occurring with children fostered by culturally inappropriate relatives or elderly and infirm people.[35] The worst-hit places are marked by intersecting, layered crises, in which the needs of orphans come on top of the demands of caring for people sick with AIDS, other adverse impacts of the disease, and other shocks and stresses such as drought and unemployment. In Kagera district of north-west

Tanzania, resilient local support networks and a relatively prosperous district economy have meant that, despite a protracted high prevalence of HIV, levels of social distress have been markedly lower.[36]

Third, are these orphans living without adequate socialization? Even in the case of the minority of orphaned children who do not have fostering arrangements, Bray argues, there is no evidence for children living outside social norms. Some children are heading households and others are living on the streets, but their resilience and determination to live within social frameworks is much more striking than any obvious anomie. Africa's striking cases of unsocialized youth and child soldiers come mostly from countries ravaged by war, usually with low HIV prevalence. As the war in Sierra Leone erupted in the early 1990s, young rebel fighters incorporated AIDS as an idiom for their angry hopelessness, justifying their extreme violence on the grounds that 'We're all going to die of AIDS anyway.'[37] At the time, rates of HIV in Sierra Leone were negligible and it is highly unlikely that any of those rural boys were infected. It was merely a metaphor, like the Liberian fighter – a Kaplanesque 'loose molecule' – who figures on the cover of Nielson's report.[38]

None of this should de-emphasize the individual needs of children orphaned by AIDS for parental affection, security and protection, schooling, an escape from poverty, health and psychosocial assistance. Orphans tend to do worse on most counts than other children, though some analysts argue that this is chiefly because they are poor.[39] Nor should it divert attention from the fact that many families are not coping but struggling, caring for orphans and the sick at the cost of their long-term livelihoods.[40]

Fourth, is this a threat to social stability? At present, an answer to this is somewhat hypothetical. Anything that impedes social and economic development is bad news, but specific links from orphans to crime and disorder are unproven. Orphans are disproportionately represented among housemaids in Addis Ababa and street children in Lusaka. But whether they are more likely to become guerrilla soldiers or gangsters is not known, and if such an association exists, it will be much more modest than the conventional predictors of conflict, notably 'war before or war next door': the brute facts of recent history of armed conflict in the country or across a border. Africa's orphans and vulnerable children should be the focus of our humanitarian concern, but the hypothesis that they will cause widespread social breakdown can be left at the margin of our worries.

The Economics of Democracy

Will AIDS jeopardize African democracies by stalling or reversing economic growth and thereby creating political crisis? This question divides into various parts: the extent and nature of the economic damage wrought by AIDS, what recession and economic restructuring mean for democracy, and whether African polities have adapted to these threats. In each case, the evidence is mixed, and an answer demands a careful look at the transformations in African democracy during the last decade.

Only one clear conclusion emerges from the debate on the economic impacts of HIV/AIDS in Africa: the economists don't know the answer. Nicoli Nattrass characterizes the understanding as 'in a rather confused state, to say the least'.[41] From a different part of the political spectrum – the IMF – Markus Haacker reaches much the same conclusion: existing models don't capture the impacts of AIDS.[42] Some models reach the intuitively distasteful conclusion that AIDS could increase GDP *per capita*, because the reduction in economic growth will be less than the reduction in population growth. This can be caricatured as the argument that Africa has surplus labour and that the disease, by reducing this surplus, will make economies function more efficiently. Others go to an opposite extreme. For example, Clive Bell and his colleagues at the World Bank have argued that, without prompt action to tackle HIV/AIDS, the South African economy could face complete collapse within four generations.[43] In the middle are some economists who refuse to include the impact of AIDS in their projections because they have yet to see a credible model for its economic impacts.[44] Nattrass points out that consensus among economic modellers is more apparent than real, because although two of three major models for the South African economy converge on similar outcomes, they do so on the basis of very different assumptions and projections. On models, she concludes, 'At best they help us think through the dynamic economic impact of AIDS. At worst they are a misleading and shaky house of cards.'[45]

There is a powerful intuitive reason for suspecting that most models understate the adverse impacts of AIDS. How is it meaningful to say that a nation's economy is growing while its citizens' life expectancy is falling? Must there not be some very important but unmeasured indicator of welfare that is crashing – perhaps the unremunerated labour of women in the home – which prefigures a plunge in the headline figure of GDP growth? If a generation is coming of age without adequate skills and values, surely 'healthy' growth rates are fragile and temporary? As we have seen: we don't know the answer and won't do so for a decade or more.

What does this mean for democracy? If we don't know what AIDS means for economic performance, we can be even less certain what its economic impacts mean for democracy. But we can still use our knowledge of how states work to build some models. What emerges is that the political context is the key, and that Africa's political systems have changed dramatically in the last decades. Rulers have sought – and often found – political protection from social dysfunction in new international support systems. 'Good governance' in Africa is sustained in part by an international consensus that there is no alternative to liberal democracy. Given African states' dependence on international goodwill and funds, this norm is not difficult to enforce.

Three hypotheses can be advanced for how AIDS-induced economic crisis could undermine democracy. The first is that economic recession itself jeopardizes democracy. This is well dealt with by Mattes and Manning,[46] who use statistical correlations to estimate that, based on their GDP *per capita*, Botswana and South Africa have 'democratic life expectancy' of 36 years, Namibia 18 years, and other southern African countries just eight years – democratic systems can only be expected to last that long under current economic circumstances. If HIV/AIDS impoverishes these countries and exposes them to economic shocks, the risks of multi-party systems failing to endure are statistically raised.[47] Predicting the longevity of political systems is only metaphorical demography: the context in which democracies survive or fail has changed markedly in the last decade. In particular, there are now a number of life-support systems for failing democracy and mechanisms for intervening when crisis intrudes. The African Union and subregional organizations have outlawed coups d'état and have acted decisively in enough cases to deter would-be putschists.

A second possibility is that the structure of economies will change. AIDS impacts economic sectors differently, depending on how vulnerable they are to the payroll tax that AIDS represents. The sectors least impacted will be minerals and foreign aid, while manufacturing and smallholder agriculture may be more vulnerable. This implies a shift away from governments with a tax base in farming and manufacturing towards rentier states relying on foreign assistance, oil and diamonds. Historically, African states that rely on these sorts of rental income have been distinctly undemocratic (with a few notable exceptions such as Botswana). Mineral revenues enable governments to raise sufficient resources without relying on a tax base among the general population and local businesses. Cold War assistance was little more than a bribe for a ruler's political loyalty, often extended precisely with a view

to insulating that ruler from the demands of domestic constituencies. The situation has changed considerably in the last 15
years. The aid encounter is often now a leverage point used by
donors to compel states to conform to norms of liberal democracy
(and market openness), at least superficially. Minerals revenue
and where it goes still remain secretive and a major locus of
corruption, but there are serious pressures for greater trans-
parency, exemplified by efforts to prohibit 'blood diamonds'.
Traditional pressures for democratic accountability exist, arising
from a tax-paying middle class seeking to constrain an arbitrary
government, but it is a changed external environment that has
made possible Africa's democratization.

It is important to be vigilant in monitoring structural changes
to African economies, and especially deepening dependency on
AIDS funds, to see how this influences democratic decision
making. International pressure has been the main factor driving
increased AIDS funding. But intensified competition for control
over incoming resources could paralyse or destabilize governments. Contests for control of AIDS funds are indeed happening,
as once-neglected ministries of health assume a new importance.
But, however well-resourced, a minister of health will never be in
the same position to make or unmake a government as his
colleague in charge of defence. Any head of state who has successfully managed his army and security services will have little
difficulty in staying on top of a well-funded and ambitious health
service.

'New Variant Famine'

A third scenario is that HIV/AIDS might unleash social crises –
such as famine – that topple governments. Of all disasters,
famines are most feared by those in power. Mass hunger brings
together a number of characteristics that make it a uniquely

serious political challenge. Famines develop over many months and are therefore never a surprise to those who go hungry, even though their rulers may have ignored the signs. The destitute congregate in towns, making famine visible and delivering the power of numbers to a political opposition ready to seize its opportunity. Perhaps most important, food is symbolically powerful and lies at the heart of customary social contracts. In most societies the failure to provide food for the starving implies a deep-rooted betrayal by the rulers. Most of those who die in famines do so through infectious diseases unleashed by the social distress that famine generates, but it is the hunger that counts politically. 'Famine' resonates in the public imaginary. This implies that an AIDS epidemic that is not itself a political threat could become one by unleashing mass hunger and distress migration.

Across sub-Saharan Africa, HIV/AIDS is impoverishing families. When a working age adult falls sick, households lose a source of income and work, and need to spend money on medication and time on care giving. Children, especially girls, may be taken out of school to work in the house or fields. Typically, families struggle to maintain their income for as long as they can, chiefly by means of the able-bodied working longer and longer hours. When an adult dies, families often sell assets to pay for funerals. Teenage daughters may be married off, partly so that the family can receive bridewealth. If it is a male head of household who has died, the widow and children may be vulnerable to losing their land and other assets to the dead man's relatives.

In an agricultural system that relies on a single rainy season and just a few labour-intensive crops, AIDS sickness and death can squeeze a family's annual seasonal labour bottleneck and quickly create a crisis. This is the situation in semi-arid savanna lands of southern Africa. The risks are further increased if the stress of the disease coincides with drought or a collapse in the market price of cash crops. In a farming system with year-round rainfall and a diversity of crops, including low-labour tree crops, families can cope better with the stresses of AIDS – as they do on the western shores of Lake Victoria, for example. Where there are strong social networks that can help an afflicted family through its most stressful period, and if the wider economy is prospering, it is much more likely that an AIDS-afflicted household can avoid destitution.

AIDS typically doesn't cause a crisis of aggregate food production. Even at the height of a generalized epidemic, the number of people who die in an affected community is too small to make anything but a marginal difference to production. And where land is the scarce factor of production, labour force losses will not mean that fields are left unfarmed. AIDS has not caused any famines. But, when a crisis strikes, households affected by AIDS are less able to cope. Households typically survive a hunger year by working harder, eating less, selling assets and calling on the assistance of relatives. All of these are more difficult or less effective when someone in the family is suffering AIDS, or there are many children dependent on fewer working adults, or relatives are already burdened by caring for orphans. Those struggling with AIDS face sharply increased handicaps on survival when food is scarce and expensive.[48] During the southern African drought of 2002–3, AIDS 'increased the depth of vulnerability of those already vulnerable to shocks…. [It] acted to intensify the disadvantages imposed on the poor.'[49] After the drought, households affected by AIDS stayed poorer and more vulnerable, and it is likely that future droughts will ratchet them down more quickly and deeply into hunger and destitution.

HIV rates in the countryside are usually lower than in the towns, but children orphaned by AIDS are often sent to rural relatives to be cared for, and adults dying of AIDS may return home to the village for their final days. Without publicly audible complaint, rural women bear the burden of the disease shifted onto them by others.

Africa's AIDS epidemic may make famine more common. It certainly makes it less tractable. The social and political profile of famine also changes with a concurrent AIDS epidemic. A traditional drought famine is geographically defined: certain areas are affected and, usually, able-bodied people will migrate from these regions to cities. One of the main political purposes of food relief distributions is to halt that migration and stop social disorder in towns. Whole constituencies are hungry: the crisis is geographically visible, it has a place name and usually a spokesman – for example, a local member of parliament, an activist or a newspaper editor. It is when rural distress wins urban champions that it becomes a political threat. By contrast, the pattern of hunger and penury that arises from AIDS is dispersed rather than concentrated, and marked by a reverse migration of the sick and orphaned from towns to villages. More like chronic poverty, AIDS-related hunger is less visible. It is also difficult to acknowledge AIDS as a cause of social distress, and harder still to politicize it.

This 'new variant famine'[50] is unlikely to translate into a political challenge to governments for one further reason. Until the 1980s, famines regularly contributed to the overthrow of African governments. Emperor Haile Selassie in Ethiopia and President Jaafar Nimeiri in Sudan are only the best-known examples. But in the last twenty years there is not a single instance of this. Governments have found ways of neutralizing this particular political threat. The parallel processes of economic and political liberalization and philanthropic globalization mean that a national government is no longer the custodian of its citizens' right to food. When people go hungry, the press and the NGO community may criticize the government, but they hold markets and international agencies such as the World Food Programme and USAID equally responsible. African rulers still resist using the word 'famine' because it reflects badly on them, but they know they can not only survive a food crisis but even use it to their advantage. Famine always had its benefits,[51] chiefly because a government is stronger when it controls the flow of life-saving resources to its people. In earlier decades, such crises were exceptional and African governments had not learned to navigate the politics of international relief. Today, extreme poverty and hunger are normal, and African governments devote much time and expertise to managing the international aid apparatus. From the host government's point of view, the main function of the aid industry is to neutralize political threats arising from social dysfunctions and to provide money. If aid reduces poverty and hunger, it is a bonus.

Rather than posing the question of its impacts as 'bad effects' versus 'no effects' it is better to consider HIV/AIDS as a subtle but far-reaching change in the trajectory of development of African polities. Although the political changes wrought by AIDS are hardly discernible today, future historians will probably point to changes that we have not even begun to recognize. Just as a mariner, setting off on an inter-oceanic voyage, who sets his compass wrongly by a single degree risks making landfall on the wrong continent, so might AIDS slowly swing Africa towards a different destiny. Nothing about this is inevitable.

We can draw some conclusions about what is happening today and what is likely in the immediate future. The socio-economic impacts of AIDS are grave, especially when layered on other crises. AIDS is sapping the human resources needed for services and development. But the fear that Africa's AIDS epidemics will sweep away its democracies is unfounded. One reason for this is that the threats of AIDS have been misrepresented. A second is that the internal structure of Africa's polities enables them to absorb most of these stresses – at a cost. And the final reason, emerging from a consideration of why famine has ceased to be a political threat, is that a disaster can always be an opportunity – especially when foreign philanthropy is at hand. The benefits of AIDS are the theme of the next chapter.

5

The Political Benefits
of AIDS

Ugandan Myths

The President of Uganda, Yoweri Kaguta Museveni, was introduced by Chinua Akukwe with these words:

> Ladies and gentlemen, Uganda beat back the deadly ravages of
> HIV/AIDS because of the courageous and principled stand of
> one individual: Yoweri Museveni. This president more than 15
> years ago decided to buck the traditional African proverb that a
> tree cannot make a forest. Mr Museveni became not only the
> proverbial tree in AIDS remedial efforts in Uganda but also
> constituted himself into a forest.... Many of us will be happy
> to save one, two, three or ten lives in our lifetime due to our
> direct actions. President Museveni has literally saved millions
> of lives in Uganda. He has also saved millions more in other
> parts of Africa by his bold, courageous and principled fight
> against HIV/AIDS.... President Museveni, you are without any
> doubt an icon and a living legend in the fight against
> HIV/AIDS in Africa.

It is customary for Africa's big men to be heralded with such flattery, and African audiences listen with practised scepticism. Akukwe was speaking in Washington DC.[1] Uganda's real story is much more interesting.

Ugandans' success in reducing their HIV/AIDS epidemic has been more celebrated than analysed. There is some good scholarship, however,[2] and there are many different explanations of why it seems to have worked. Most AIDS analysts see it as a combination of enlightened leadership by Museveni and a practical application of a range of policies, including what became known as the 'ABC' approach,[3] openness and multi-sectoral programming. At the Bangkok AIDS conference in July 2004, Museveni explained the 'ABC': 'Abstain from sex or delay having sex if you are young and not married, Be faithful to your sexual partner (zero grazing), after testing, or use a Condom properly and consistently if you are going to move around.'[4] But it is a mistake to see Uganda's AIDS policies as a 'best practice' of international orthodoxy. In fact, the approach was innovated in the 1980s at a time when 'best practice' had yet to crystallize, and derives in large part from the wider political practice and philosophy of the National Resistance Movement. Later, and in an unexpected and *ad hoc* way, AIDS has become integral to Museveni's strategy for wielding power.

If we judge Museveni's actual record on AIDS against the 'best practice', it is wanting in several respects. To start with, Museveni has not been open with the figures. He has overstated the decline in prevalence, claiming in 2000 for example that national prevalence had come down from 30 per cent in 1991 – a figure that is probably twice as high as the reality. The Ugandan official response to any questioning of these figures is scathing and intimidating. After Justin Parkhurst wrote that 'the importance of the Ugandan experience will be compromised if conclusions are drawn out of context and statements are made on the basis of oversimplified assessment of epidemiological data',[5] he was pilloried by government ministers who not only insisted that the President's figures were fully scientific, but imputed that non-African critics were motivated to play down African success.[6] Major Rubaramira Ruranga is also sceptical of the government claims: 'We should stop producing doctored information for fear of evaluation and for want of more money.'[7] Conversely, Museveni has played up his role in bringing about the success: 'The decline these people are talking about was because I went around preaching in every county, that is why there was a dramatic fall.'[8] Any leader seeks to capitalize on success. What is surprising is that Museveni's claims are so often taken at face value.

Ugandans have more mixed opinions about their president than the international consensus might suggest. While the majority approve of the government AIDS policy, Afrobarometer data also show a significant critical constituency. Those who prioritize AIDS the most are also the most critical of the government, a pattern that resembles South Africa's. It is also instructive to compare Tanzania and Kenya, which have a broadly similar (though more recent) pattern of HIV prevalence rise and decline, yet have not been celebrated in the same way.

Museveni is famous for his openness in talking about AIDS. He has the demeanour of a charismatic preacher or teacher, who uses humour to talk about sensitive issues such as sex. In the early days, Museveni spoke directly to the Ugandan people. At the end of the 1990s, he began to trumpet his success and use it for political credit – perhaps because his military involvement in Congo was becoming politically costly and the country's long economic boom was coming to an end.[9] At the African Development Forum, held at the United Nations Economic Commission for Africa in Addis Ababa in 2000, he recounted his triumphs and said, 'most important of all, the stigma attached to people living with HIV/AIDS has virtually evaporated'. But alongside this tolerant affability, from the outset he has also conveyed a different, tougher message that doesn't match up to the rhetoric of overcoming stigma. This message, consistently purveyed, is that his army and government cannot afford to invest in people with HIV. 'The army is not a hospital,' Museveni said, explaining why he did not promote soldiers who tested positive for HIV. Some Ugandan AIDS activists were outraged at his remarks at the passing-out ceremony for newly commissioned army cadets in April 2001, in which he said 'there is no reason why people living with HIV/AIDS should be offered opportunity in the army. Because training officers who later die not from bullets in combat but from AIDS is so frustrating. It is like fetching water in a basket with holes.'[10] At the same ceremony eighteen months later, the government newspaper reported how he cautioned the cadets against 'reckless and immoral sexual behaviour'.[11] As well as 'ABC' his approach has an implicit 'D': discipline.

The former guerrilla has given variants of the story of how he was alerted to the scale of his AIDS problem. One episode often recurs, namely how after taking power Museveni sent 60 National Resistance Army officers to Cuba for training: the Cubans routinely tested them for HIV, and 18 were positive. The NRA was not only Museveni's power base, it was the base from which he intended to pursue revolutionary transformation. On taking the oath of office, the new president said he intended 'no mere change of guards but a fundamental change'. But according to his Marxist analysis, all the major pillars of a dependent bourgeois state remained: an unreconstructed police, judiciary and bureau-cracy, as well as parasitic and dependent economic élites. Only the army and the Resistance Councils were committed to the revolution. One of Museveni's senior officers, Ondoga ori Amaza, wrote: 'Rather than marking the end of the NRA's bush war, the 1986 NRA capture of power only set the stage for continuation of the war by other means.'[12] How was this ongoing revolution to be accomplished if the vanguard was dying? Five years earlier, the NRA's guerrilla war had been launched by a tiny *foco* of 27 armed men, led by Museveni, who attacked Kabamba barracks in

western Uganda. The mythologized 'Kabamba 27' were in fact
nearly forty – a dozen more did not have weapons. In 1995,
Ondoga traced 37 of them. Seven had been killed in the guerrilla
war, three had died in subsequent wars (two in Rwanda), and one
had died in a motorcycle accident. Of the remaining 26, eight had
died of illnesses between 1988 and 1995, and two were dead of
unknown causes, leaving just 16 survivors. Disease had claimed
more than the liberation war. Ondoga himself (not one of the 37)
died of illness before he could see his book published. It is
suspected that Lyantonde, home town to many close relatives of
the ruling élite, suffers an especially high rate of HIV.[13]

In Uganda, politics is an extension of the military. In 2001,
when challenged in the presidential election by his former
colleague-in-arms, Dr Kizza Besigye, Museveni alleged that his
rival could not run the country because he 'has AIDS'.[14]
Museveni's allegation is unproven, but the claim that a man living
with HIV should not lead the nation or command the army is
perfectly consistent with his expressed views. As commander-in-
chief of the Ugandan People's Defence Force (successor to the
NRA as the national army), Museveni oversees the lists of the
officers who receive ART. This is both an exercise in triage and the
ultimate form of patronage. One doctor who had worked with
the army said, 'if one sees the list of beneficiaries of Museveni's
authorization for treatment, it becomes difficult to avoid accusing
him of nepotism'.[15]

ABC: Carefully Mixed Messages

The ABC formulation gives Museveni plenty of opportunity for
tailoring his message to his audience. He is not being incon-
sistent: he wants different people to behave differently, and he
also wants different things from different audiences. In his early
awareness campaigns, Museveni told girls in élite secondary

schools that if they had to eat sweets, they should do so with the wrapper on. Around the same time, he also spoke of condoms as 'at best, a short-term solution. What works is a change in behaviour ... the whole problem is tied in with the breakdown of morals in the world.'[16] Puritanism is often found alongside revolutionary militancy. Some years later, he made an international audience laugh by saying, with emphasis, 'next year we shall require eighty million condoms!' Meanwhile the President berates rural leaders for promoting condoms – attacking condom distributions in primary schools, for example. 'I am going to review this issue. I will open war on the condom sellers. Instead of saving life they are promoting promiscuity among young people.'[17] Revealingly, he continued: 'When I proposed the use and distribution of condoms, I wanted them to remain in town for the prostitutes to save their lives.' A few months later Museveni repeated the message, adding, 'I have grown-up children and my policy was to frighten them out of indisciplined sex.'[18] A laudatory editorial in the government-owned *New Vision* newspaper explained that 'one memorable analogy the President has used in illustrating how one can avoid HIV infection is that of a person who keeps on poking fingers into every hole in anthills and ultimately gets beaten [sic: bitten] by a snake'.[19]

President Museveni and his wife Janet carefully size up their foreign audiences. International opinion was not important when Uganda's AIDS efforts were launched twenty years ago. Home-grown and largely domestically funded for the first few years, Uganda's AIDS programme has since grown massively in size and repute. When HIV incidence in Uganda began to fall, just a few million dollars had been spent. That turnaround became an invaluable asset a decade on, providing a political cachet of growing value. Janet is a born-again Christian and her message goes down well in conservative circles in Washington DC: 'Giving young people condoms is tantamount to giving them a licence to be promiscuous; it leads to certain death.'[20] The Bush administration is not only funding Uganda's AIDS programme through the President's Emergency Program for AIDS Relief (PEPFAR) but is a political ally of the increasingly isolated Ugandan leader. In a different context, Janet's husband has continued his long-standing criticism of the Roman Catholic church for prohibiting condoms: 'This is not to support immorality, but to recognize the weakness of those we live with and help them to live a healthy life.'[21]

However, Ugandans see a clear shift in their President's messages. Influenced by his wife and by the US agenda of abstinence-only AIDS programmes, in the last two years he has emphasized the 'AB' and downplayed the 'C'. To the dismay of AIDS activists and practitioners, government policy has shifted sharply against condoms, which the government is reluctant to procure and distribute.

These different emphases make sense when we analyse the national AIDS programme and how it has evolved. Just a few months after taking power, in May 1986, the Minister of Health told the World Health Assembly in Geneva that the country was facing an AIDS epidemic. The initial response was medical: the government set up an AIDS Control Programme. Later on, a multi-sectoral AIDS programme was launched, headquartered in the President's Office. This became an exemplar of 'leadership' and 'mainstreaming.' It was also about power. The NRA's revolution was driven from a single power centre – the presidency, which also served as the high command for the army – and all the institutions of government needed to be transformed and made subservient to it.

Note the word 'control': the AIDS Control Programme was also a mechanism for social control and mobilization within a leftist tradition of revolutionary warfare. In this tradition, members of the vanguard have privileged access to knowledge and are permitted to debate different opinions within their own circle, in order to arrive at the correct analysis. The masses have no such opportunity for thinking for themselves and must simply follow the 'correct line' mapped out for them. Such a philosophy melds neatly into patrimonial governance. During the armed struggle, the NRA was famous both for its child soldiers – known as *kadogos* – and for the discipline and effectiveness of those children. A sympathetic commander could provide a surrogate father figure for the *kadogos* in his care, while an undisciplined one would neglect his charges and expose them to danger.[22] In the liberated areas, the 'Resistance Council' system was a Leninist-style organizational hierarchy which also meshed with local power structures – sometimes old ones, sometimes new. They were seamlessly transformed into the new administrative system after the NRA took power and are to this day the bedrock of Museveni's constituency. Among the tasks of Resistance Councils were controlling and constraining young people's social and sexual intercourse. This began as part of the social discipline needed to conduct a people's war and was readily adapted to AIDS control measures. For example, they would stop young women moving from village to village and close down discos and bars. In areas thought to be politically antagonistic, this included threats and violence against women whose behaviour was considered socially unacceptable. Sorcery accusations – with the concomitant threat of lynching – were also made against some women who were thought to be potential spreaders of HIV. Just as central government extended its authority into rural areas through the Resistance Councils, so the Councils exerted their authority over young people and especially young women.[23]

The extent of coercion in rural Uganda – and in some other instances of successful behavioural change – is rarely acknowledged. To do so would be considered distasteful or even dangerous. The Ugandan government, AIDS NGOs and international AIDS policy makers prefer to sustain the fiction that all behavioural change is purely voluntary. There are distinct ethical and instrumental cases for voluntariness and an *a priori* argument for respecting individual human rights as paramount. There is an argument, ably advanced by Jonathan Mann among others, that AIDS can only be tackled and overcome by gaining the active consent and support of everyone who is at risk or infected. This is part of a wider shift in public health strategies in developed countries, away from control-based measures towards placing responsibility on the individual.[24] Its efficacy depends on other parallel social changes, including high levels of health awareness, a climate of liberal individualism and, most important of all, universal access to good-quality health services. Where these conditions are lacking, the principle of voluntariness is less meaningful and can become an excuse for failing to acknowledge and deal with the social structures that determine behaviour.

The acceptability and success of coercive measures was hugely helped by the economic rebound after the end of the war, including the revitalization of the rural economy, the opening of schools and the return of émigrés. Museveni's smartest move was to return property to the Ugandan Asians who had been expelled by Idi Amin in 1971: the investment that they brought in far outstripped any levels of foreign aid that Uganda has received then or since, and provided a massive quick injection of productive capital into the economy.

In the cities, by contrast, Museveni allowed a limited liberalization. Alongside the hierarchical one-party system, he permitted uncensored newspapers and a proliferation of NGOs. While rural people were expected to conform to 'traditional' moral discipline, urban people were instructed to 'love carefully'. The distinct approaches reflect the Leninist theory of the national democratic revolution as a staging post on the road to a true socialist revolution, a tactical compromise with the bourgeois élites needed to keep the country running. So, bourgeois values were permitted in the towns, and members of the revolutionary vanguard were allowed to debate freely, but the peasantry and proletariat – the true revolutionary power base – were to be protected from such subversive influences. Over time, Museveni's revolutionary ambitions became submerged within stratagems focused on remaining in power. Like many liberation leaders in government, his energy and ideals dissipated, but the centralized political-military nexus of power remained intact along with undiminished militaristic commitment to crushing his opponents.

The Ugandan AIDS Commission was established in the Office of the President in 1992, and it prepared a 'Multi-sectoral Approach to the Control of AIDS' the following year. AIDS policy makers saw this as the beginning of a model strategy for overcoming AIDS. For Museveni, however, this was the culmination: no more was needed. The strategy document – redrafted several times at considerable expense – has stayed on Museveni's desk. It has not become law. AIDS activists and practitioners complain that this lack of legislative authorization is a major hindrance to their efforts. For Museveni, it means he keeps absolute discretionary authority, and, as noted by Major Rubaramira, the UAC loyally 'propagates the achievements of President Museveni and portrays a picture of government commitment'.[25] Museveni would like all his government departments to function that way.

Another nexus between AIDS and power in Uganda is the budget. As well as controlling the guns, the President needs to control the money. This led in 2003 to controversy over health spending. Uganda, as a highly indebted poor country, has agreed with its foreign creditors on an economic strategy based on restraining government spending, controlling inflation and thereby seeking to encourage saving and attract foreign investment, as a means for economic development and poverty reduction. The IMF and World Bank support this approach, which is enforced by Uganda's finance ministry. The ceiling on the Ministry of Health's spending was US$107 million. In 2003, Uganda was awarded a grant by the Global Fund of US$52 million over three years. The grant application was completed by the Minister of Health, who considered this the minimum

Table 5.1. Sectoral shares of Uganda's national budget allocations (%)[26]

Year	Defence/security	Health	Education
1996	18.3	7.4	21.8
1997	16.2	7.2	22.7
1998	17.4	6.6	24.6
1999	18.7	6.7	27.8
2000	14.0	7.3	24.9
2001	12.1	9.0	24.2
2002	12.9	9.6	24.9
2003	14.3	9.5	22.9

necessary for scaling up the country's AIDS programme. The grant would have catapulted health spending through the expenditure ceiling, and the Ministry of Finance duly responded by instructing the Ministry of Health either to refuse the grant, to scale it back, or to take the money but return other health funds to the treasury – thereby making the grant spurious. Charles Wendo, the journalist following the story, noted that 'the Ministry of Finance has fixed a ceiling below the floor'.[27] Activists accused the IMF of sticking to inflation targets in a doctrinaire manner, regardless of human cost. After protracted negotiations, a compromise was reached whereby the grant was scaled down somewhat, stricter controls were placed on its usage, but AIDS spending was placed outside the government's overall fiscal framework. But in 2004, when the publicity storm had quietened, the *status quo* was resumed.

This controversy is usually cited as an example of a government that wanted to spend money on its AIDS programme but was unable to do so because of IMF strictures. There is no doubt that the IMF approved of capping spending. But the key decisions came from the Ministry of Finance in Kampala. It imposed the ceiling, relaxed it under pressure from AIDS lobbies, and then re-imposed it in the following year. Table 5.1 shows budgetary allocations in Uganda. This is an incomplete record because health and education consistently underspend their budgets while defence and security overspend, and also because significant parts of the defence and security sector spending are extra-budgetary (especially given that Ugandan forces have twice invaded Congo during this time). Nonetheless it shows the trends.

There have been improvements in the balance of spending over the past ten years. Universal primary education is one of Museveni's most popular policies and the education budget is robust. But health spending has not increased commensurately with its official prioritization, while defence spending has decreased only modestly. The real villain in this piece is not the IMF; it is the allocation to the military.

Yoweri Museveni has come a long way since he and his small band of comrades opened fire at Kabamba. He stormed the citadel of state power and gained legitimacy by bringing peace, stability and relative prosperity to most of the country. But his second decade in power has been marred by foreign wars, corruption and an increasingly despotic style of government. He has kept the single-party system (it is officially a 'no-party' system) and changed the constitution to allow him to continue running for office indefinitely. European and American governments no longer like to deal with leaders who do such things. In these circumstances, Museveni's greatest asset is his AIDS 'success story' – exaggerated but real nonetheless. The international community needs this one success, and Museveni knows it, and he and his wife know how best to explain it to different audiences. Museveni's rule has lost most of its sources of legitimacy, save the mythology around AIDS.

'Fighting' AIDS

Uganda under Museveni is an odd mixture of liberalism and militarism, as is the country's AIDS effort. The language of AIDS policy reflects the president's fondness for military metaphors: he promises to 'crush' both his opponents and socio-economic problems alike. For activists and political leaders, it seems almost impossible to avoid using the language of war when dealing with crime, illiteracy or any other social ill. Typically, a 'war' on corruption will involve the selective targeting of middle-ranking officials and an occasional senior politician, each of them singled out for reasons of political convenience. The overall system of corruption will not be touched. In a 'war' on poverty or illiteracy, the presidency will bypass the standard government departments with a special taskforce. It is unlikely that sustainable gains will follow. The main long-term result will be to strengthen the power of the chief executive *vis-à-vis* the bureaucracy.

At the opening of the African Development Forum on leadership and AIDS in December 2000, a parade of dignitaries made fighting speeches.[28] Dr Salim Ahmed Salim, Secretary General of the Organization of African Unity, opened the Forum by saying, 'There is a dire need to reorient the concept of national security to transcend the invasion of borders and threats to government.... Our societies, in their entirety, have to enter into a combat mode for liberating themselves from the pandemic.'[29] The then head of the UN Development Programme, Mark Malloch Brown, vowed to put his agency 'on a war footing' to defeat AIDS. The Ethiopian President Negasso Gedada described HIV/AIDS as 'a national disaster that needs an even greater level of national mobilization than that devoted to armed conflict'. He went on to promise that, having just concluded a conventional war with Eritrea, Ethiopia would now mobilize itself for a 'war against AIDS'.

The only speaker in that eminent parade who had experience of a shooting war – Graça Machel, who had served in Mozambique's liberation struggle – avoided the masculine imagery of war fighting.[30] She preferred to talk about the need for respecting and involving women and girls and changing men's values: 'Some of our communities continue to educate young men with notions of manhood that encourage them viewing having multiple partners as natural and normal.... In this era of HIV/AIDS, different priorities must be developed and different values exemplified by our young men.'

The African Development Forum consensus document called for new finance for AIDS in Africa, a funding drive comparable to the Jubilee 2000 campaign to abolish debt. The call was repeated four months later at a special summit of African nations held in Abuja, Nigeria, on AIDS, tuberculosis and other related infectious diseases – the latter added mainly to appease Thabo Mbeki. From that conference was born the Global Fund *to Fight* AIDS, TB and Malaria (emphasis added), created by the UN a few months later.

Metaphors can be useful for cultural critique and political polemic. As Salim implied, could the military metaphor be refined to refer to more than a liberation war against an occupying power? In such a case, the kind of effort required would not be repelling an invader at the border but mobilizing people's warriors to win back control of occupied territory. This usage has more depth, but it is still a metaphor. Could the somewhat ludicrous 'declarations of war' be turned back on their originators in an exercise of mockery and calling to account? If the three speakers cited above were all generals, surely their losses in the following years would have led them to be cashiered.[31] The only one still in office – Malloch Brown, now promoted to be the UN Secretary-General's chief of staff – can be challenged on his record. But he is a soft target, as the whole audience in Addis Ababa, despite their applause, knew he didn't really mean it.[32] 'About that metaphor, the military one,' Susan Sontag concludes, better to 'give it back to the warmakers.'[33]

Museveni, like many African leaders, is indeed a war maker, to whom the metaphor comes instinctively. It usefully emphasizes the values of discipline, obedience, nationalism and masculinity. While these traits may not serve the cause of 'fighting' AIDS particularly well, they are the routine imagery of state power.

This is how governments behave, using any public policy issue to increase their resources and advance their authority. It is a means of acknowledging a threat and domesticating it. Those in the 'front line' – health workers, volunteers and ordinary people providing care for the sick and orphaned children – instinctively distrust the military metaphor and don't use it. 'War' on AIDS has more to do with the supposed warriors than their proclaimed struggle. It signals an attempt to continue business as usual. While African and international civil society organizations strive to situate AIDS efforts within a liberal rights framework, heads of state try to recapture those programmes as militaristic exercises.

On the Difficulties of Showing Success

Perhaps the most important and least surprising lesson from Uganda's story is that it tells us a lot about Uganda but not much about anywhere else. The 'Ugandan success story' is a bundle of paradoxes, explicable only within the country's particular history. Museveni has run a one-party state for twenty years, while tolerating an independent media and civil society. About half his national budget is derived from foreign aid, but he has succeeded in navigating the politics of international donors and retaining considerable latitude to pursue his interests – notably confounding international orthodoxy by repeatedly postponing multi-party elections and serially invading neighbouring countries. Above all he has been adept in manipulating the emergent structures of global AIDS governance to his advantage. Museveni responded adroitly to AIDS, but not because of Ugandan public opinion. Meanwhile the decline in HIV prevalence is more to do with what ordinary Ugandans did for themselves than with any government leadership.

Uganda also shows that it takes a very long time to reverse an HIV/AIDS epidemic. In their thorough appraisal of the evidence,

Daniel Low-Beer and Rand Stoneburner estimate that new HIV infections (incidence) began to decrease in 1988. In about 1992, prevalence levels (the proportion of people living with HIV, irrespective of when they were infected) peaked and by 1994 national surveillance was marking its first measurable decline.[34] This was recognized the following year in Rakai and Masaka and soon afterwards in other locations – when Uganda first began getting recognition as a 'success story'.[35] The numbers of people dying from AIDS follows the incidence curve, about eight to ten years later, so that AIDS deaths hit their peak in 1996–8.[36] The number of children newly orphaned by AIDS tracks the AIDS death curve but the total number of orphans will have continued to rise for five to seven years more.[37] Returning to the beginning – the incidence reduction – we don't know how far in advance changes in sexual behaviour began, in order for them to feed through into fewer infections. Let us assume, quite arbitrarily, that it took two years, which implies that behavioural changes began in 1986. Those changes took about 17 years or so to work through their major human impacts. And it was only half-way through this process (in about 1994) that there was any measurable success – the first reported declines in prevalence.

Eight years to show the first signs of success, and a further nine to pass the peak of human impact – that is an impossibly long time for an elected politician or a career civil servant to reap rewards. Museveni has been in power throughout the entire period and is doing his best to stake his claim. But two terms in office, four or five years each, is the norm, and for good reason. A scenario project by UNAIDS noted how the 'trap of swift dividends', symptomatic of low trust societies, makes it difficult to mount the requisite long-term AIDS control programmes.[38] A newly elected president who succeeds in 'getting it right' on AIDS will see his successor, or his successor's successor, preside over the turnaround. This assumes, of course, that AIDS 'best practices' actually work – an assumption with rather little evidence to support it. Botswana implemented an AIDS education programme at the same time as Uganda with the same components and a comparable or higher level of commitment. From that date, Botswana's response has been a model. But over more than fifteen years it has had no measurable impact on HIV prevalence, which rose from an estimated 5 per cent in 1990 to 18 per cent in 1992 and 36 per cent in 2002. Prevalence has now stopped rising, but that plateau may be as much due to the internal dynamics of the endemic – reaching saturation levels – as to any government activities.

Measuring success is technically complicated. The key indicator for success in prevention efforts is HIV incidence. This has been hard to measure (though technical advances in testing are making it much easier) and is not in fact monitored anywhere consistently. As a proxy, leaders say that things are getting worse when prevalence rates go up, and claim the credit for success when they go down. But prevalence estimates vary for many reasons, including the death rate of people with HIV (as people live longer with ART, prevalence rates will increase), migration and – the commonest reason of all – methodological changes in the way of collecting and analysing data. One can understand why Ugandan health officials were frustrated when their claims of success were challenged by a British PhD student.[39]

A better way of measuring success in HIV prevention would not only be a useful tool for statisticians and health planners. It would also provide a shorter-turnaround reward for politicians. The right information is essential for creating the necessary political incentives for responding to AIDS. Until there is a reliable measure of HIV incidence, democratic governments will have one more reason for not increasing their level of political commitment to tackling HIV/AIDS. It is instructive to compare how developed countries respond to the threats of SARS and avian flu by setting up incidence monitoring systems with extremely rapid reporting schedules.

A disturbing lesson emerges from this analysis. We have not measured success in overcoming HIV/AIDS within a time frame that matches the political calendar. Without this, the political incentives for *really tackling HIV transmission* – as opposed to *being seen to follow approved practices* – are weak. Our analytical models and evidence base are inadequate, which leaves the door open for the opportunistic exploitation of fragments of good news for political ends. It is disappointing that, two decades into Africa's epidemic, we should still be in this position.

Treatment Regimes

Given the structural difficulties with prevention policies, it is unsurprising that foreign donors and AIDS activists have made treatment their priority, and governments are moving in that direction too. Antiretroviral treatment has a natural constituency: people living with HIV and AIDS and their families, friends and employers. Doctors like it too. It is a measurable service with clear and quite rapid pathways from inputs to outcomes. It is a tangible means of managing the socio-political risks of the epidemic, by keeping people alive. These considerations mean that ART serves well as a focus for activist mobilization and political reward. But treatment also has hazards.

Taking ART to scale is the most ambitious service delivery exercise ever undertaken in Africa. It poses an array of formidable challenges: much higher levels of testing, building health infra-structure and especially training and retaining the required number of health workers, meeting the nutritional, shelter, and liveli-hoods needs of patients, ensuring patient compliance and correct use of drugs, and monitoring drug-resistant strains. It requires formidable discipline in a health system and a population. Moreover all this must be done with a very modest evidence base for what might work and scant attention to the sad history of failed grand schemes for saving Africa. Operations research is pitifully funded and what little is being conducted is occurring in parallel with the scale-up of treatment. ART roll-out is a huge social experiment conducted in real time.

Treatment's incentive structure is the converse of prevention's: results can be demonstrated in a few years, but the risks emerge down the line. The biggest biomedical danger is that strains of HIV resistant to first-line drugs will emerge. There are already disturbing stories of antiretrovirals being retailed with minimum medical supervision or shared with other HIV-positive family members without prescription or monitoring. Many hospitals have 'cash and carry' windows where drugs, including ARVs, are dispensed. There are political risks, too, as ART scale-up poses immense ethical and public policy challenges.

These controversies begin with testing. The norm for HIV testing is shifting from being purely voluntary to making testing part of routine medical examination. Botswana is leading the way on this. The near-universal practice of mandatory testing in African armies, which is considered unethical according to UN standards, is being discreetly adopted as standard.

Best-practice standards for treatment access are still evolving. They include medical criteria, gender equality and some consideration of the value of the individual – the needs of medical staff and mothers are often highlighted. It is a fudge typical of liberal-NGO governance: all are equal but some more so than others. In a positive light, it is an example of the civil society–AIDS apparatus setting a high ethical bar that national treatment programmes probably will approach over time. More interesting for our analysis is the political sociology of an ethically reflective non-universal treatment roll-out.

Uneven ART provision is literally rationing the right to life. If it is not done transparently, rationing will be done quietly and implicitly.[40] In a developed country with high and articulate demands for medical equity, such rationing would generate political outcry. Some have voiced the fear that it will create political crisis in Africa.[41] It is certainly easy to imagine people living with HIV and AIDS staging public demonstrations to dèmand treatment available to others and denied to them. But at present that is not happening. Is this another intriguing instance of apparent political quiescence by African publics in the face of disaster and injustice? Or is it that powerful constituencies have quieter but no less effective methods for staking their claim to treatment? Probably it is a bit of both. People living with HIV and AIDS are rarely an organized constituency and not, as we have seen, a revolutionary one. Groups such as army officers and senior civil servants make sure they get the treatment they demand without the need to make adversarial claims in public.

Treatment rationing is a fact. Only in Africa's richest and best-governed states – South Africa, Botswana and Namibia – is there any prospect of the state providing universal treatment. But even here, a patchwork approach to treatment access is emerging – a combination of explicit and implicit rationing. Some private sector employers provide ART to their staff, perhaps after restructuring so that low-paid tasks are now subcontracted out, along with responsibility for those workers' health care. Better-off individuals themselves obtain treatment from private clinics. Government institutions – especially the army – quietly provide for their own. NGOs do likewise, often with the support of their donors. Some of these programmes extend to family members. For the majority, an uneven array of public clinics, NGO services and churches serves as an ART delivery system. The real criteria for rationing depend on access to these sources of funds and influence – an ad hoc system reflecting the way in which the African state has been cannibalized by various interest groups, including donors, corporations, its own power brokers and NGOs.[42] In some respects it resembles a patrimonial system. In other respects, it is a form of reconstituted statehood in which citizens have a range of different entities to which they can appeal, none of which commands all of the sovereign space, and which between them only provide for a minority of the people living in a particular territory.

This inequitable system is being established with little public debate and less political outcry. Is this because AIDS is still not seen as a public political issue? Because the actual demand for ART is still far smaller than the potential demand, for the reason that so many people do not know their status or are in denial? Or because African citizens have such low expectations of their governments?

Even with reduced drug prices, treatment is expensive and requires a lot of trained people and superb organization. Some activists have worried that the focus on treatment is detracting from prevention. This is, broadly speaking, unlikely to happen. Unprecedented amounts of money are flowing into HIV/AIDS activities, and testing and treatment programmes all contribute to public education and hence (it is assumed) prevention. Of more concern is the fear that treatment provision will consume the continent's scarce human and infrastructural resources and thereby crowd out other essential tasks. There is a high opportunity cost to treatment provision, which may be seen in other parts of the health sector, or in education and other services. On the other hand, the funds flowing into employment in ART roll-out should help to stimulate local economies.

Funds for AIDS programmes have expanded from 2 per cent to 10 per cent of Africa's official development assistance between 2001[43] and 2004,[44] and are still growing. Global AIDS funding has grown from US$1 billion in 1999 to over US$8 billion in 2005. If projections are realized, aid for AIDS could amount to as much as a third of Africa's aid by the end of the decade. At present, about 80 per cent of Africa's HIV/AIDS programmes are financed from international sources, and that proportion is certain to rise as pledged monies come on-stream. This may create a wholly new model for African governance in which a dominant function of national governments and NGOs is to serve as a mechanism for processing donor funds to provide ART to keep people alive.

A state that is so highly dedicated to extending the lives of its citizens is, in principle, social democratic in the extreme and based on a strong social contract. Nicoli Nattrass concludes her book *The Moral Economy of AIDS in South Africa* with these words:[45]

> AIDS is different because it is a public health crisis, which not only has deep social roots, but challenges the very notion of what it means to be a society. Serious social reflection and debate will not only help raise the consciousness of citizens about AIDS (thereby contributing to prevention), but will shape a genuine social response to this challenge. AIDS policy is too important to be left to the technocrats.

Only in a few cases does the national government have the resources and capacity to attend to this task itself. South Africa is one of these exceptional cases, and the politics of mobilization around AIDS in that country might just produce a social contract of this nature. Elsewhere, it is improbable. Sub-Saharan Africa's biggest-ever service delivery operation is being implemented with a multiplicity of new actors, with massive infusions of foreign funds and expertise, and in governing systems that are often neo-patrimonies. We are on the brink of an unparalleled life-controlling intrusion into African societies, and we just don't know what it will look like.

Treatment trials and NGO pilot projects have shown that Africans can have excellent treatment compliance rates, but participants in trials are carefully selected and NGO micro-projects cannot easily be replicated at scale. Achieving the necessary compliance rates and monitoring systems will require an un-paralleled level of intrusiveness and discipline. Governments will be tempted to advocate coercion, but they lack both the means and the political licence to exercise it.

Alongside the welfarist social contract, three other scenarios for a society dominated by ART provision can be drawn in carica-ture. The first we can call the 'grassroots democracy provides

ART' model, in which there is a profusion of civil society initiatives, enabling African society to meet this challenge from the bottom up. Scenario two is the 'citadel of expertise'. Following the historic pattern of scientific medicine in Africa, governments and donors will create a remote, bureaucratic and distrusted apparatus. It will struggle with its own norms and procedures, making modest improvements but forever shackled by unmet goals and frustrated ideals. As the AIDS apparatus becomes ever more concerned with its internal workings, democracy will be compromised and dependency deepened. The third scenario is 'coopted by patrimonialism', in which traditional-style African despotisms reproduce their paralytic centralism in the field of ART, channelling first-rate medical care to those in power and ignoring the rest.

Each of these scenarios is likely to be present in differing configuration in each African country. In each case, the most powerful actors will be able to ride out the stresses of the HIV/AIDS epidemic, keeping their power intact and adjusting their structures and strategies according to changing circumstance. We have seen how one African leader has been able to do this to his notable advantage. Others have been neither so skilled nor so lucky, but they are learning. International organizations and local NGOs are similarly learning to adjust to HIV/AIDS, taking advantage of new resource flows and opportunities for influence. Huge public policy decisions are being taken in an *ad hoc* manner. The shortage of evidence brings advantages to the most powerful: they can tell their version of the story without fear of refutation and embark upon policies designed to further their interests.

Two major questions remain. Will the governance mechanisms that emerge promote democracy and human rights? And will they succeed in overcoming HIV/AIDS, or will treatment roll-out simply become the best mechanism for managing the risks of AIDS, a substitute for prevention measures? These are the concern of the final chapter.

6

Power, Choices and Survival

Lutaaya, 'Alone'

Philly Bongole Lutaaya sang his greatest song about dying of AIDS. In 1989, the Ugandan singer was the first famous African to declare his status. He continued performing while visibly sick, touring the country with his song 'Alone', which implored people living with HIV and AIDS to 'come on out, let's stand together, fight AIDS, in times of joy, in times of sorrow.... With open hearts, let's stand up and speak out to the world.' After Lutaaya died in December that year, the video film of his last concerts, *Born in Africa*, became a bestseller.

Lutaaya is unique among mainstream musicians in bluntly using the word 'AIDS' in his lyrics. He dressed his theme in fighting imagery familiar to Ugandans, who had just emerged from civil war, massacre and dictatorship. By doing so, he placed this new, invisible and bewildering virus in the public imagination of Ugandans. This was vital: we need to *imagine* HIV/AIDS before we can think practically about it. Lutaaya made AIDS into news, which made ordinary people talk about AIDS in buses, bars, marketplaces and churches.

Lutaaya's imagery of 'standing together' to 'fight' AIDS reso-
nated among Ugandans who had stared collective oblivion in the
face just a few years before, during the darkest days of the Idi
Amin and Milton Obote governments when it seemed as though
the country would become little more than a graveyard marked
by pyramids of human skulls. The singer's call for sacrifice and
renewal was more than rhetoric for audiences who had seen their
houses pillaged and their families killed or forced to flee, and had
picked up a hoe and started again. All this they had done without
foreign help and scarcely with international acknowledgment: the
Ugandan massacres of the early 1980s, the defining episode in
that country's history, are still strangely absent from Africa's
historical archive.

Seventeen years on, Lutaaya is still alone in his openness about
AIDS. So, too, is Uganda in its striking success in reversing the
climb of HIV, following changes in sexual behaviour in the late
1980s. By the time Lutaaya went on his last tour, his audiences
had *already* seen AIDS and they were *already* reducing the number of
sexual encounters in which HIV was transmitted. Daniel Low-
Beer and Rand Stoneburner comment:

> The first international lesson out of Uganda, is that the response
> preceded and exceeded HIV interventions. Ugandans managed
> their epidemic, took credit for success, and national and
> international policy provided support, rather than the other way
> around. HIV policy and prevention started in these villages, and
> political and public health interventions built on this.[1]

It is sobering to reflect on the fact that Africa's best-known
'success story' began before the inflow of international aid for
AIDS, before the national AIDS policies were adopted, before
Museveni's famed speeches, and even before Lutaaya's song. It
should give us even more pause for thought to reflect that, almost
twenty years on, HIV prevalence is falling in only a few countries.
We don't know much about preventing HIV.

In Chapter 2 we analysed how public figures such as Lutaaya created AIDS as a news item, which in turn translated into public discussions on the topic, in due course changing public attitudes. But this does not explain why President Museveni adopted 'best practice' AIDS policies. He did that for his own political reasons. Government policy, public attitudes and NGO activism are all important in their own right, but do not explain why HIV rates began to fall in Uganda. This was happening already. Most likely, there are links between public attitudes, activism, government policies and sexual behaviour. We just don't know what they are.

Democracies Can Manage AIDS

The analysis in this book has posed more questions than it has answered. The dynamics of the HIV/AIDS epidemic and its impacts are not well understood, and the processes whereby societies become energized to respond effectively to AIDS are equally mysterious. We know much more about the rapidly changing socio-political context in which AIDS has struck Africa, and how responses to AIDS operate.

Some conclusions can be reached with confidence. The most important of these is that the HIV/AIDS epidemic itself does not threaten African political systems. Governments and institutions are designed to handle threats to their survival, and HIV/AIDS has turned out to pose a political threat no greater than familiar pathologies such as hunger and homelessness. AIDS has been politically domesticated. Anti-retroviral treatment has become the central mechanism for managing AIDS, but even before treatment scale-up began a few years ago, governments and international agencies had proved adept at managing the risks emanating from the disease. Encouragingly, Africa's democratization is protected from the impact of AIDS, because participation and human rights are embedded not only in citizens' aspirations but also in new international norms, and because the response to the AIDS epidemic has itself been enmeshed in these norms. Rulers and policy makers who prefer to 'fight' AIDS in an authoritarian manner have so far not succeeded in recapturing AIDS efforts. They may have more success as the demand for ART increases in parallel with AIDS budgets and efforts to ensure discipline in treatment compliance.

AIDS struck Africa while a hybrid form of democracy was emerging on the continent. It is plausible that the social and economic conditions of political and economic transition, including population mobility and the relaxation of old social norms, actually expedited the spread of HIV. That is a subject for a different book. What is relevant here is that Africa's new democracies are characterized by the diffusion of power and influence throughout international institutions and the increased permeability of these institutions to activism by élite civil society. The aid machine, formerly an obstacle to accountability, is now promoting participation. But as the aid apparatus grows in size and power, its nature could change. The march to democracy can always be stalled, reversed or distorted by donor country interests or by militarized patrimonialism. Alongside the aspirational model of citizen as partner, Africa still possesses deeply embedded patriarchal forms of political legitimacy and control. Projects for direct control of the populace, such as dictatorships and armed liberation struggles, continually re-emerge.

The international AIDS apparatus has been in the vanguard of democratizing the aid encounter. AIDS activists have been instrumental in promoting an agenda of AIDS response based on voluntary participation and human rights, rather than on control. In turn, activists have become powerful players within international AIDS organizations. As treatment expands, the AIDS apparatus is growing extremely fast and its character will change. It could become a mechanism for raising a host of neglected issues and giving some influence to voiceless groups. AIDS activism could spark challenges to the equally shameful neglect of mass poverty and absence of social welfare in Africa – chronic hidden scandals in themselves, that would not be tolerated in any developed country. But, equally, international AIDS organizations could also solidify into an introverted bureaucracy that soldiers on, pushing certain formulae on African societies. Across Africa, people suspect that coercion is lurking, and retain a deeply embedded resistance to external citadels of expertise and their projects of extending bureaucratic power. The future AIDS response may be part of a project of liberalization-through-aid, but equally it could become another doomed-to-fail foreign intrusion or a prop to authoritarianism, an ally of the war-making approach to AIDS efforts.

In the next few years, public policy decisions of immense import will be taken that will determine which course is taken. Because the evidence and analysis are so scarce, ideology and interest will mainly determine what choices are made. With the right political mobilization, African democracies can not only survive AIDS but actually become stronger.

Democracies Do Not Prevent HIV

The response to AIDS in Africa has achieved many things. It has protected the rights and influence of AIDS constituencies and ensured that norms of human rights and participation are observed. It has informed tens of millions of Africans about HIV/AIDS and is providing treatment to several hundred thousand. What it has not done is prevented HIV transmission itself. The epidemic is largely unchecked. There are reports of lower HIV prevalence in a number of countries (most recently Kenya and Zimbabwe) and among certain demographic groups. But we don't know if this is the outcome of different measurement methods, social and epidemiological changes associated with the path of the epidemic, or AIDS policies and programmes. Given the controversies surrounding the Ugandan experience, it is understandable that governments and many AIDS organizations prefer not to look too closely.

The international AIDS effort could succeed in its aims. The funds now available could make the difference. Well-funded prevention and treatment programmes could work, and welfare assistance could bring millions of AIDS-affected families out of poverty. But many things could also go deeply awry. The experiment in treatment at scale could collapse or backfire. Prevention strategies have not worked to date and there is no guarantee that they will in the future.

Governments and institutions don't know how to reduce HIV infections and are not subjected to political pressures and incentives to make them learn. While in 25 years scientists have learned more about the human immunodeficiency virus than about any other pathogen, we still lack solid evidence and analysis on what public health measures work and why. We measure viral load in an individual but not new HIV infections in a population. We know very accurately the effects and side-effects of ARVs but we have no idea whether decades' worth of AIDS education messages have any impact at all. Equally surprising is the low level of motivation to compile the evidence and undertake the analysis: there is an assumption that we know enough and just need to try harder. The prematurely achieved and unobjectionable consensus that is the stock-in-trade of international agencies is an obstacle to the kinds of inquiry and debate that are necessary. This book has tried to show that good social scientific research routinely confounds the accepted wisdom and reveals a more complicated, interesting and often unexpected picture.

There are some signs of change: more resources, better technology and stronger activist mobilization. But there are also formidable obstacles to making real efforts to overcome HIV/AIDS a public policy priority. One important obstacle is 'constructive denial'—the maintenance of a false normality.

Another is a premature policy consensus based on poor evidence and analysis. But these can be overcome. Critical social science research will certainly challenge some of the shibboleths that continue to dominate the field of AIDS. A free and well-informed press, not afraid of uncertainty and controversy, is the most important tool for generating the kind of public discussion that can lead to political engagement. Only with much better evidence and information will it be possible to create real political incentives to which governments and international organizations might respond. Only then will it be possible for African nations to face the momentous public policy decisions forced on them by AIDS, and decide in an informed and democratic way.

The fundamental lesson, unsurprising to anyone familiar with the history of social engineering and foreign aid in Africa, is that AIDS efforts are driven ultimately by institutional and political interests. As individuals, AIDS policy makers often have the highest motives and great insight, and work exceptionally hard. Individuals can make a difference, but their institutions are almost as intractable as the epidemic itself. The iron laws of institutions routinely subvert the best intentions. Default mode for governments and institutions is to secure their own survival and they are doing very well on this score. They are prolonging lives through treatment. But they are doing miserably in terms of preventing new HIV infections, because they haven't been required to succeed. When African and international electorates punish their leaders for this failure, we can expect progress.

We have every reason to be angry. AIDS will not prove the political calamity that some have feared. It shows no sign of bringing about revolution, anarchy or terrorism, and it is unlikely to threaten the global order. But HIV/AIDS is a human tragedy on an awful scale, and there is no end in sight. As Susan Sontag writes, 'That even an apocalypse can be made to seem part of the ordinary horizon of expectation constitutes an unparalleled violence that is being done to our sense of reality, to our humanity.'[2]

Notes

Chapter 1

1   Caldwell 1997, p. 180.
2   'We Are All Threatened by This Plague', *International Herald Tribune*, 29 July 2005. Laurie Garrett's article mistakenly located the incident (discussed in Chapter 3) in Cape Town.
3   <www.lauriegarrett.com>.
4   One national action framework for coordinating partners' actions, one national AIDS coordinating authority, and one country-level monitoring and evaluation system.
5   For the mathematics of this, see Blacker and Zaba 1997.
6   Roman Rollnick, 'Botswana's High-stakes Assault on AIDS', *Africa Recovery*, 16, 2–3 (2002).
7   Afrobarometer 2004a.
8   Whiteside *et al.* 2003.
9   Afrobarometer 2004b, p. 5.

Chapter 2

1   Afrobarometer 2004a, p. 1.
2   Edwin Cameron compares scientific denialism to revisionist historians

who deny that the Nazi Holocaust of European Jews occurred. See Chapter 4 and Cameron 2005, pp. 131–49.

3   Samantha Willan, preparatory research for this book.

4   Willan 2004b, p. 11.

5   Afrobarometer 2004b, p. 5.

6   Cohen 2001, pp. 7–8.

7   <www.queerme.com.aids>, accessed 8 June 2005.

8   CNN, 'Falwell Apologizes to Gays, Feminists, Lesbians', 14 September 2001.

9   Cf. Patton 1986.

10 Badri 1997, p. 210.

11 In line with a particular strand of Islamist thinking known as Bucaille-ism, which claims that the Qur'an and Hadith contain the essence of all modern scientific discoveries (and therefore could only have been dictated by the Almighty), he interprets the Prophet's words to antici-pate viral mutation.

12 Mbilinyi and Kaihula 2000.

13 Ibid., p. 87.

14 Kelly 2004.

15 Cf. McGuire 2003, who notes that secular scholars of world-ending events do not anticipate this privilege.

16 HIV is a slow-acting retrovirus in the lenti-virus class.

17 Cohen 2001, pp. 6–7, 128, 138.

18 Daniel 2005.

19 Schatzberg 2001.

20 Mbembe 2001.

21 H. Campbell 2003, pp. 124, 131.

22 World Bank 1999, pp. 57–76.

23 Ibid., p. 75.

24 Morris and Kretzschmar 1997; Halperin and Epstein 2004.

25 Caldwell et al. 1989.

26 Heald 2003.

27 Another of the Caldwells' favoured themes – that male circumcision protects against HIV transmission – was also disregarded for many years until recent evidence demonstrated dramatically lower HIV risk among circumcised men.

28 Mahamud-Hassan 2004.

29 Mandisa 2005.

30   Luirink 1998, pp. 21–2.

31   ter Haar and Ellis 2004.

32   Ashforth 2005.

33   Ibid., p. 69.

34   Evans-Pritchard 1937.

35   This too harks back to the academic ancestors of social anthropology, such as Meyer Fortes.

36   Ashforth 2005, p. 70.

37   Desmond *et al.* 2004.

38   Ibid., p. 48.

39   Cliggett 2005, Chapter 6. However, Elizabeth Colson earlier noted that funeral costs had not increased.

40   C. Campbell 2003.

41   Wallman 1996.

42   Ashforth 2005, p. 280.

43   Sontag 1988.

44   Gould 1987.

45   Afrobarometer 2004b, p. 5. This holds when controlling for any correlations between media access and HIV risk.

46   Sample size: N = 23,197.

47   Bor 2005. As measured by the 'political support' score of the AIDS Program Effort Index (The POLICY Project, UNAIDS, USAID).

48   See also Wendo 2003.

49   Wendo 2003, p. 15.

50   Analysis by Jacob Bor.

51   Dow 2000.

52   Andreas 2001.

53   Mpe 2001.

54   Ibid., p. 18.

Chapter 3

1   Modise Kabeli, 'Ministry "Not Aware" of Shots Fired at Activists', <www.dispatch.co.za/2005/07/16/easterncape/act.html> accessed 9 September 2005.

2   TAC press release, 'Forty Injured, Ten Shot at Peaceful Protest to Demand Treatment', 13 July 2005.

3   See Heywood 2005.

4   Zackie Achmat, 'HIV/AIDS and Human Rights: a New South African Struggle', 2004 John Foster Lecture, 10 November 2004.

5   Ballard 2005, Gumede 2005, pp. 279–88.

6   Abraham 2003.

7   Manning 2002, p. 6.

8   Willan 2004b, p. 10.

9   Bor 2005.

10 Strand 2005.

11 The following paragraphs on this topic are drawn directly from her work. See Willan 2004a, 2004b.

12 Strand 2005, p. 3.

13 Willan 2004a, pp. 109–117

14 Department of Health, 2003, Operational Plan for Comprehensive HIV and AIDS Care, Management and Treatment for South Africa, <www.health.gov.za>, p. 52.

15 *TAC Newsletter*, 26 July 2004, 'Monitoring Report of ARV Roll Out', <www.tac.org.za>.

16 Quinlan and Willan 2005.

17 Kramer 1983.

18 Kramer 1989.

19 Global AIDS Alliance 2002.

20 Dalton 1989.

21 Epstein 1997.

22 <http://www.irinnews.org/AIDSreport.asp?ReportID=1700>, accessed 17 October 2005.

23 <http://www.ahfgi.org/global_pdf/UNAIDS.pdf>, accessed 17 October 2005.

24 Cameron 2005, pp. 131–49.

25 De Cock and Johnson 1998.

26 *Ibid.*, p. 290.

27 De Cock, Mbori-Ngacha and Marum 2002, pp. 68–9.

28 Baldwin 2005, pp. 128–9.

29 Whiteside, de Waal and Tsadkan 2006.

30 Baldwin 2005.

31 Vaughan 1991.

32 Feierman 1990.

33 Ferguson 1994.

34   Leach and Mearns 1996.

35   McCulloch 2002.

36   Aké 1995.

37   *Ibid.*, p. 79.

38   Mbembe 2001, p. 36.

39   Saunders 1999.

40   Keck and Sikkink 1998, pp. 12–13.

41   Cf. Habib 2005.

42   Cf. Lieven 2004, p. 63.

43   Shilts 1987.

44   Garrett 1994, 2000, 2005.

45   Behrman 2004.

Chapter 4

1   de Waal 2003.

2   McPherson *et al.* 2000.

3   See also Mattes and Manning 2004.

4   Mattes 2003.

5   Strand 2005.

6   Independent Electoral Commission, <www.elections.org.za>.

7   'Special Voting Arrangements', media release, 25 March 2004, <www.elections.org.za/news.>

8   Speaking to the author, November 2005.

9   Manning 2003.

10   *Ibid.*, p. 22.

11   *Ibid.*, p. 17.

12   Strand *et al.* 2005, p. 18.

13   De Waal 2003; Mattes and Manning 2004, p. 211.

14   Similar objections can be made to the 'Adam Smith in reverse' hypothesis.

15   Chabal and Daloz 1999; van der Walle 2001, Bayart, Ellis and Hibou 1999; Mbembe 2001; Schatzberg 2001.

16   Pritchett 1999.

17   Ostergard and Tubin 2004; Elbe 2003.

18   Whiteside, de Waal and Tsadkan 2006.

19   Rana 2004, p. 56.
20   Schatzberg 2001.
21   Schaffer 1998.
22   Schönteich 2000.
23   Pharoah 2004.
24   Urdal 2004.
25   Kaplan 1994. This is sometimes labelled a 'Lord of the Flies' scenario after the William Golding novel.
26   Neilson 2005, pp. 4–5.
27   See Amnesty International's report on the Democratic Republic of Congo, in which these claims are made. According to AI, children have been 'repeatedly' obliged to carry out atrocities, 'some' were forced to kill their families and 'others have been made to engage in cannibalistic or sexual acts with the corpses of enemies killed in battle' <http://web.amnesty.org/ library/index/engafr620342003>.
28   The rationale for wearing women's clothing and other extravagant dresses is rather more complex. See Ellis 1999.
29   AIDS has created thousands of households headed by children, almost all of them teenagers. There are reports of individual households headed by younger children, usually because continuing to reside in the homestead retains the household's land rights.
30   Islamic Jihad and other similar organizations operate in countries with very low rates of HIV and the AIDS epidemic is a minor part of their cosmology and ideology (see Chapter 2). In sub-Saharan Africa there are very few child terrorists. The best-cited cases are RENAMO in Mozambique, the Lord's Resistance Army in Uganda, and Liberian factions, but even in these instances conspicuous atrocities by young child combatants were exceptional, if peculiarly tragic and well-publicized.
31   Bray 2003.
32   de Waal 2004.
33   Madhavan 2003.
34   de Waal et al. 2004.
35   Nyambedha, Wandibba and Aagaard-Hansen 2003.
36   There is a rich literature documenting HIV/AIDS and its impacts in Kagera. The most recent information comes from a ten-year follow-up cohort study conducted by Economic Development Initiatives. See de Weerdt 2001.

37   Richards 1999.
38   The picture was taken by Chris Hondros of Getty Images, and is described thus: '"Exultant Commander" – MONROVIA, LIBERIA – JULY 20: A Liberian militia commander loyal to the government exults after firing a rocket-propelled grenade at rebel forces at a key strategic bridge July 20, 2003 in Monrovia, Liberia. Government forces succeeded in forcing back rebel forces in fierce fighting on the edge of Monrovia's city center.' <www.nppa.org/competitions/best_of_still_photojournalism/2004/winners/still/MAN> accessed 20 June 2005. UNAIDS estimated HIV prevalence in Liberia at 5.9 per cent of adults in 2003, and 36,000 of the country's 230,000 orphans were orphaned by AIDS.
39   Crampin *et al.* 2003, Lindblade *et al.* 2003.
40   The phrase comes from Rugalema 2000.
41   Nattrass 2004, p. 160.
42   Haacker 2004a, 2004b.
43   Bell, Devarajan and Gersbach 2004.
44   Ali Abdel Gadir Ali, personal communication 2002.
45   Nattrass 2004, p. 162.
46   Mattes and Manning 2004.
47   *Ibid.*, pp. 194–5.
48   de Waal and Whiteside 2003, de Waal 2006.
49   Wiggins 2005, p. 11.
50   de Waal and Whiteside 2003.
51   Cf. Keen 1994.

Chapter 5

1   Luncheon organized for President Museveni by the Pharmaceutical Research and Manufacturers of America, Constituency for Africa, Africa Society of the National Summit on Africa and Church World Service, 12 June 2003, Washington DC.
2   See especially Allen and Heald 2004, Allen 2006.
3   The 'ABC' acronym originated in Botswana and was used in Uganda later on. See Allen 2006.
4   Yoweri Museveni, 'Behavioral Change is the Only Way to Fight AIDS',

Wall Street Journal, 14 July 2004.
5   Parkhurst 2002, p. 78.
6   Charles Wendo, 'UNAIDS Chief Defends Uganda on AIDS Story', *New Vision*, 9 July 2002.
7   Interviewed by Kintu Nyago for this book.
8   Oluput and Maseruka 2004.
9   Tumushabe 2005.
10 Tshihamba 2001.
11 Jonathan Angura, 'Museveni Advises Cadets on AIDS', *New Vision* (Kampala), 11 November 2002.
12 Ondoga ori Amaza 1998, pp. 148–9.
13 Tumushabe 2005.
14 Marguerite Michaels, 'Three is a Crowd in Love and Politics', *Time*, 12 March 2001.
15 Tumushabe 2005.
16 Speech dated 1992, in compendium of speeches, cited in: Institute for Youth Development 2002.
17 Eddie Ssejoba, 'Museveni Condemns Condom Distribution to Pupils', *New Vision* (Kampala), 17 May 2004.
18 Oluput and Maseruka 2004.
19 Editorial, 'Museveni Correct on Condom Limits', *New Vision* (Kampala), 16 July 2004.
20 Janet K. Museveni 2004; Peter Gill, 'Experts Attack Bush's Stance in AIDS Battle', *Observer* (London), 11 July 2004.
21 UN IRIN (Integrated Regional Information Network) 2005.
22 Rabwoni 2002.
23 See Allen 2006.
24 Baldwin 2005.
25 Interviewed by Kintu Nyago for this book.
26 Source: Ministry of Finance, Planning and Economic Development, Republic of Uganda.
27 Wendo 2002, p. 1847.
28 UNECA 2001.
29 *Ibid*.
30 Museveni spoke at the closing session.
31 One is reminded of the celebrated headline in the satirical newspaper *The Onion*: 'Drugs win drug war.'
32 At the closing session of the Forum, a panel of heads of state was

challenged on why Africa spent more money on war than AIDS. While Meles Zenawi and Yoweri Museveni justified their military actions, Botswana's President Festus Mogae humbly admitted that 'we have failed' – and then said that no effort should be spared to bring peace to Africa.

33 Sontag 1988, p 183.
34 Low-Beer and Stoneburner 2004.
35 Allen 2006.
36 The peak of AIDS mortality in the mid-1990s may be a substantial part of the reason why HIV prevalence fell dramatically at that time.
37 The precise pattern depends upon the definition of 'orphan' and whether it includes children up to 15 or up to 18.
38 UNAIDS 2005, pp. 116–17.
39 Parkhurst 2002.
40 Rosen *et al.* 2004.
41 Cheek 2001.
42 Cf. Reich 2002.
43 OECD and UNAIDS 2004, p. 21.
44 UNAIDS 2004.
45 Nattrass 2004, p. 189.

Chapter 6

1 Low-Beer and Stoneburner 2004, p. 182.
2 Sontag 1988, p. 134.

Bibliography

Abraham, Curtis (2003) 'Angel of Africa', *New Scientist*, 8 March.

Achmat, Zackie (2004), 'AIDS and Human Rights: a New South African Struggle', 2004 John Foster Lecture, 10 November.

Afrobarometer (2003) 'Freedom of Speech, Media Exposure, and the Defence of a Free Press in Africa', Afrobarometer Briefing Paper No. 7, July.

—— (Michael Bratton, Carolyn Logan, Wonbin Cho and Paloma Bauer) (2004a) 'AfroBarometer Round 2: Compendium of Comparative Results from a 15-Country Survey', Afrobarometer Working Paper No. 34.

—— (2004b) 'Public Opinion and HIV/AIDS: Facing Up to the Future?' Afrobarometer Briefing Paper No. 12, April 2004.

Aké, Claude (1995) 'The Democratisation of Disempowerment in Africa', in Jochen Hippler (ed.), *The Democratisation of Disempowerment: the Problem of Democracy in the Third World*, London: Pluto.

Allen, Tim (2006), 'AIDS and Evidence: Interrogating Some Ugandan Myths', *Journal of Biosocial Science*.

Allen, Tim and Suzette Heald (2004) 'HIV/AIDS Policy in Africa: What Has Worked in Uganda and What Has Failed in Botswana?' *Journal of International Development*, 16, 8: 1141–54.

Altman, Dennis (1988) 'Legitimation through Disaster: AIDS and the Gay Movement', in Elizabeth Fee and Daniel M. Fox (eds.), *AIDS: the Burdens of*

History, Berkeley: University of California Press.

Andreas, Neshani (2001) *The Purple Violet of Oshaantu*, Oxford: Heinemann.

Angura, Jonathan(2002) 'Museveni Advises Cadets on AIDS', *New Vision* (Kampala), 11 November.

Ashforth, Adam (2005) *Witchcraft, Violence and Democracy in South Africa*, Chicago: University of Chicago Press.

Badri, Malik (1997) *The AIDS Crisis: an Islamic Socio-Cultural Perspective*, Kuala Lumpur: International Institute of Islamic Thought and Civilization.

Baldwin, Peter (2005) *Disease and Democracy: the Industrialized World Faces AIDS*, Berkeley: University of California Press.

Ballard, Richard (2005) 'Social Movements in Post-Apartheid South Africa: an Introduction', in Peris Jones and Kristian Stokke (eds.), *Democratising Development: the Politics of Socio-Economic Rights in South Africa*, Leiden: Martinus Nijhoff Publishers.

Bayart, Jean-Francois, Stephen Ellis and Beatrice Hibou (1999) *The Criminalization of the State in Africa*, London: James Currey.

Baylies, Carolyn (2002) 'The Impact of AIDS on Rural Households in Africa: a Shock Like Any Other?' *Development and Change*, 33: 611–32.

Behrman, Behr (2004) *The Invisible People: How the US Has Slept through the Global AIDS Pandemic, the Greatest Humanitarian Catastrophe of Our Time*, New York: Free Press.

Bell, Clive, Shantayanan Devarajan and Hans Gersbach (2004) 'Thinking about the Long-run Economic Costs of AIDS', in Markus Haacker (ed.), *The Macroeconomics of HIV/AIDS*, Washington DC: International Monetary Fund.

Blacker, John and Basia Zaba (1997) 'HIV Prevalence and Lifetime Risk of Dying of AIDS', *Health Transition Review*, 7 (Supplement 2): 45–62.

Bor, Jacob H. (2005) 'The Politics of National Responses to AIDS in Developing Countries', undergraduate thesis, Harvard University.

Bray, Rachel (2003) 'Predicting the Social Consequences of Orphanhood in South Africa', University of Cape Town, Centre for Social Science Research, Working Paper No. 29.

Caldwell, John C. (1997) 'The Impact of the African AIDS Epidemic', *Health Transition Review*, 7 (Supplement 2): 169–88.

Caldwell, John C., Pat Caldwell and P. Quiggin (1989) 'The Social Context of AIDS in Sub-Saharan Africa', *Population and Development Review*, 37, 8:185–234.

Cameron, Edwin (2005) *Witness to AIDS*, London: I. B. Tauris.

Campbell, Catherine (2003) *Letting Them Die: Why HIV Prevention Programmes Fail*, London: International African Institute and James Currey.

Campbell, Horace (2003) *Reclaiming Zimbabwe: the Exhaustion of the Patriarchal Model of Liberation*, Cape Town: David Philip.

Chabal, Patrick and Jean-Pascal Daloz (1999) *Africa Works: Disorder as Political Instrument*, London: James Currey.

Cheek, Randy (2001) 'Playing God with HIV: Rationing HIV Treatment in Southern Africa', *African Security Review*, 10, 4.

Cliggett, Lisa (2005) *Grains From Grass: Ageing, Gender and Famine in Rural Africa*, Ithaca: Cornell University Press.

Cohen, Stan (2001) *States of Denial: Knowing about Atrocities and Suffering*, London: Polity.

Crampin, C. *et al.* (2003) 'The Long-term Impact of HIV and Orphanhood on the Mortality and Physical Wellbeing of Children in Rural Malawi', *AIDS*, 17.

Dalton, Harlon L. (1989) 'AIDS in Blackface', *Daedalus* (1989), reprinted in Chris Bull (ed.), *While the World Sleeps: Writing from the First Twenty Years of the Global AIDS Plague*, New York: Thunders Mouth, 2003.

Daniel, Marguerite (2005) 'Beyond Liminality: Orphanhood and Marginalisation', unpublished paper, University of East Anglia.

De Cock, Kevin M. and Anne M. Johnson (1998) 'From Exceptionalism to Normalisation: a Reappraisal of Attitudes and Practice around HIV Testing', *British Medical Journal*, 316: 290–3.

De Cock, Kevin M., Dorothy Mbori-Ngacha and Elizabeth Marum (2002) 'Shadow on the Continent: Public Health and HIV/AIDS in Africa in the Twenty-first Century', *The Lancet*, 360: 67–72.

de Waal, Alex (1997) *Famine Crimes: Politics and the Disaster Relief Industry in Africa*, London: International African Institute and James Currey.

—— (2003) 'How Will HIV/AIDS Transform African Governance?' *African Affairs*, 102: 1–24.

—— (2004) *Famine that Kills: Darfur, Sudan*, Oxford: Oxford University Press.

—— (2006) 'AIDS, Hunger and Destitution: Theory and Evidence for the "New Variant Famine" Hypothesis in Africa', in Stephen Devereux (ed.), *The New Famines*, forthcoming.

de Waal, Alex and Alan Whiteside (2003) '"New Variant Famine": AIDS and Food Crisis in Southern Africa', *The Lancet*, 362: 1234–37.

de Waal, Alex, Joseph Tumushabe, Masuma Mamdani and Blandina Kilama (2004) 'Changing Vulnerability to Crisis in Tanzania: Implications for

Children and UNICEF Activities', report to UNICEF Tanzania, September.

de Weerdt, J. (2001) 'Community Organisations in Rural Tanzania: a Case Study of the Community of Nyakatoke, Bukoba Rural District', Bukoba: Economic Development Initiatives (EDI), February.

Department of Health (2003) 'Operational Plan for Comprehensive HIV and AIDS Care, Management and Treatment for South Africa', <www.health.gov.za>.

Desmond, Christopher, John King, Jane Tomlinson, Conway Sithungo, Nina Veenstra and Alan Whiteside (2004) 'Using an Undertaker's Data to Assess Changing Patterns of Mortality and their Consequences in Swaziland', *African Journal of AIDS Research*, 3, 1: 43–50.

Dow, Unity (2000) *Far and Beyon'*, San Francisco: Lute Books.

Drèze, Jean (1990) 'Famine Prevention in India', in J. Drèze and A. Sen (eds.), *The Political Economy of Hunger, Vol. II: Famine Prevention*, Oxford: Clarendon Press.

Elbe, Stefan (2003) *Strategic Implications of HIV/AIDS*, London: International Institute for Security Studies, Adelphi Paper 357.

Ellis, Stephen (1999) *The Mask of Anarchy: Roots of Liberia's Civil War*, London: Hurst.

Epstein, Steven (1997) 'AIDS Activism and the Retreat from the "Genocide" Frame', *Social Identities*, 3, 3: 415–39.

Evans-Pritchard, Edward E. (1937) *Witchcraft, Oracles and Magic Among the Azande*, Oxford: Clarendon Press.

Feierman, Steven (1990) *Peasant Intellectuals: Anthropology and History in Tanzania*, Madison: University of Wisconsin Press.

Ferguson, James (1994) *The Anti-politics Machine: Development, Depoliticization and Bureaucratic Power in Lesotho*, Twin Cities: University of Minnesota Press.

Garrett, Laurie (1994) *The Coming Plague: Newly Emerging Diseases in a World Out of Balance*, New York: Farrar, Strauss and Giroux.

—— (2000) *Betrayal of Trust: the Collapse of Global Public Health*, Westport, CT: Hyperion Press.

—— (2005) 'We Are All Threatened by This Plague', *International Herald Tribune*, 29 July.

Gill, Peter (2004) 'Experts Attack Bush's Stance in AIDS Battle', *Observer* (London), 11 July.

Global AIDS Alliance (2002) 'Turning Their Backs on Africa: President George W. Bush and G7 Countries Fail to Confront Global AIDS Genocide', press release, 25 June.

Gould, Stephen Jay (1987) 'The Terrifying Normalcy of AIDS', *New York Times Magazine*, 19 April.

Gumede, William M. (2005) *Thabo Mbeki and the Battle for the Soul of the ANC*, Cape Town: Zebra Press.

Haacker, Markus (2004a) 'HIV/AIDS: the Impact on the Social Fabric and the Economy', in Markus Haacker (ed.), *The Macroeconomics of HIV/AIDS*, Washington DC: International Monetary Fund.

—— (2004b) 'The Impact of HIV/AIDS on Government Finance and Public Service', in Markus Haacker (ed.), *The Macroeconomics of HIV/AIDS*, Washington DC: International Monetary Fund.

Habib, Adam (2005) 'The Politics of Economic Policy-Making: Substantive Uncertainty, Political Leverage, and Human Development', in Peris Jones and Kristian Stokke (eds.), *Democratising Development: the Politics of Socio-Economic Rights in South Africa*, Leiden: Martinus Nijhoff Publishers.

Halperin, Daniel and Helen Epstein (2004) 'Concurrent Sexual Partnerships Help to Explain Africa's High HIV Prevalence: Implications for Prevention', *The Lancet* (3 July): 4–6.

Heald, Suzette (2003) 'The Absence of Anthropology: Critical Reflections on Anthropology and AIDS Practice in Africa', in George Ellison, Melissa Parker and Catherine Campbell (eds.), *Learning from HIV and AIDS*, Cambridge: Cambridge University Press.

Hewitt, Kenneth (1983) 'The Idea of Calamity in a Technocratic Age', in Kenneth Hewitt (ed.), *Interpretations of Calamity, from the Viewpoint of Human Ecology*, Boston MA: Allen and Unwin.

Heywood, Mark (2005) 'Shaping, Making and Breaking the Law in the Campaign for a National HIV/AIDS Treatment Plan', in Peris Jones and Kristian Stokke (eds.), *Democratising Development: The Politics of Socio-Economic Rights in South Africa*, Leiden: Martinus Nijhoff Publishers.

Hunter, Susan (2003) *Black Death: AIDS in Africa*, New York: Palgrave Macmillan (also published in London by Palgrave Macmillan under the title *Who Cares: AIDS in Africa*).

Hutchinson, Janis (2003) 'HIV and the Evolution of Infectious Diseases', in George Ellison, Melissa Parker and Catherine Campbell (eds.), *Learning from HIV and AIDS*, Cambridge: Cambridge University Press.

Institute for Youth Development (2002), *Uganda: Building Blocks of Hope: the ABCs of HIV/AIDS*, Washington DC: IYD, December.

Kaplan, Robert (1994) 'The Coming Anarchy', *Atlantic Monthly*, February.

Keck, Margaret and Kathryn Sikkink (1998) *Activists Beyond Borders: Advocacy*

Networks in International Politics, Ithaca: Cornell University Press.

Keen, David (1994) *The Benefits of Famine: a Political Economy of Famine and Relief in Southwestern Sudan 1983–89*, Princeton: Princeton University Press.

Kelly, M. J. (2004) 'The Case for the Condom', *Index on Censorship*, 1/04: 80–3.

Kramer, Larry (1983) '1,112 and Counting', reprinted in Chris Bull (ed.), *While the World Sleeps: Writing from the First Twenty Years of the Global AIDS Plague*, New York: Thunders Mouth, 2003.

—— (1989), 'Equal to Murderers', in 'Reports from the Holocaust: the Making of an AIDS Activist', 1989, reprinted in Chris Bull (ed.), *While the World Sleeps: Writing from the First Twenty Years of the Global AIDS Plague*, New York, Thunders Mouth, 2003.

Leach, Melissa and Robin Mearns (eds.) (1996) *The Lie of the Land: Challenging Received Wisdom on the African Environment*, London: International African Institute and James Currey.

Lieven, Anatol (2004) *America Right or Wrong: an Anatomy of American Nationalism*, Oxford, Oxford University Press.

Lindblade, K. A. *et al.* (2003) 'Health and Nutrition Status of Orphans <6 Years Old Cared for by Relatives in Western Kenya', *Tropical Medicine and International Health*, 8: 67–72.

Low-Beer, Daniel and Rand Stoneburner (2004) 'Uganda and the Challenge of HIV/AIDS', in Nana Poku and Alan Whiteside (eds.), *The Political Economy of AIDS in Africa*, Aldershot: Ashgate.

Luirink, Bart (1998) *Moffies: Gay Life in Southern Africa*, Cape Town: David Philip.

Madhavan, Sangeetha (2003) 'Fosterage Patterns in the Age of AIDS: Continuity and Change', *Social Science and Medicine*, 58: 1443–54.

Mahamud-Hassan, Nimco (2004) 'It Doesn't Happen in Our Society', *Index on Censorship*, 1/04: 38–41.

Manning, Ryann (2002) 'The Impact of HIV/AIDS on Civil Society. Assessing and Mitigating Impacts: Tools and Models for NGOs and CBOs', Durban: Health Economics and AIDS Research Division.

—— (2003) 'The Impact of HIV/AIDS on Local-level Democracy: a Case Study of the eThekweni Municipality, KwaZulu-Natal, South Africa', Democracy in Africa Research Unit, CSSR Working Paper, No. 35.

Mattes, Robert (2003) 'Healthy Democracies? The Potential Impact of AIDS on Democracy in Southern Africa', Institute for Security Studies, Working Paper No. 71.

Mattes, Robert and Ryann Manning (2004) 'The Impact of HIV/AIDS on Democracy in Southern Africa: What Do We Know, What Do We Need to Know, and Why?' in Nana Poku and Alan Whiteside (eds.), The Political Economy of AIDS in Africa, Aldershot: Ashgate.

Mbali, Mandisa (2005) 'The Treatment Action Campaign and the History of Rights-Based, Patient-Driven HIV/AIDS Activism in South Africa', in Peris Jones and Kristian Stokke (eds.), Democratising Development: the Politics of Socio-Economic Rights in South Africa, Leiden: Martinus Nijhoff.

Mbembe, Achille (2001) On the Postcolony, Berkeley: University of California Press.

Mbilinyi, Marjorie and Naomi Kaihula (2000) 'Sinners and Outsiders: the Drama of AIDS in Rungwe', in Carolyn Baylies and Janet Bujra (eds.), AIDS, Sexuality and Gender in Africa, London: Routledge.

McCulloch, Jock (2002) Asbestos Blues: Labour, Capital, Physicians and the State in South Africa, Oxford: James Currey.

McGuire, Bill (2003) A Guide to the End of the World: Everything You Never Wanted to Know, Oxford: Clarendon Press.

McPherson, Malcolm, Deborah Hoover and Donald Snodgrass (2000) 'The Impact on Economic Growth in Africa of Rising Costs and Labor Productivity Losses Associated with HIV/AIDS', JFK School of Government, Harvard, August.

Michaels, Marguerite (2001) 'Three Is a Crowd in Love and Politics', Time, 12 March.

Morris, Martina and Mirjam Kretzschmar (1997) 'Concurrent Partnerships and the Spread of HIV', AIDS, 11, 5: 681–3.

Mpe, Phaswane (2001) Welcome to Our Hillbrow, Pietermaritzburg: University of KwaZulu-Natal Press.

Museveni, Janet K. (2004) Address by Her Excellency Janet K. Museveni, First Lady of the Republic of Uganda, Conference on 'Common Ground: A Shared Vision for Health', hosted by the Medical Institute for Sexual Health, Washington DC, 17–19 June.

Museveni, Yoweri (2004) 'Behavioral Change Is the Only Way to Fight AIDS', Wall Street Journal, 14 July.

Nattrass, Nicoli (2004) The Moral Economy of AIDS in South Africa, Cambridge: Cambridge University Press.

Neilson, Trevor (2005) 'AIDS, Economics and Terrorism in Africa', Global Business Coalition on AIDS, January.

Nyambedha, E. O., S. Wandibba and J. Aagaard-Hansen (2003) 'Changing

Patterns of Orphan Care Due to the HIV Epidemic in Western Kenya', *Social Science and Medicine*, 57: 301–11.

OECD and UNAIDS (2004) 'Analysis of Aid in Support of HIV/AIDS Control, 2000–2002', Paris and Geneva: Organization for Economic Cooperation and Development and Joint United Nations Programme on HIV/AIDS.

Oluput, Milton and Josephine Maseruka (2004) 'Museveni Opposes Condoms in Schools', *New Vision* (Kampala), 30 November.

Ondoga ori Amaza (1998) *Museveni's Long March from Guerrilla to Statesman*, Kampala: Fountain Press.

Ostergard, Robert and Matthew Tubin (2004) 'Between State Security and State Collapse: HIV/AIDS and South Africa's National Security', in Nana Poku and Alan Whiteside (eds.), *The Political Economy of AIDS in Africa*, Aldershot: Ashgate.

Parkhurst, Justin (2001) 'The Crisis of AIDS and the Politics of Response: the Case of Uganda', *International Relations*, 15: 69–87.

—— (2002) 'The Ugandan Success Story: Evidence and Claims of HIV-1 Prevention', *The Lancet*, 360: 78–80.

Patton, Cindy (1986) *Sex and Germs: the Politics of AIDS*, London: Black Rose Books.

Pharoah, Robyn, (ed.) (2004) *A Generation at Risk? HIV/AIDS, Vulnerable Children and Security in Southern Africa*, Pretoria: Institute for Security Studies.

Power, Samantha (2002) *A Problem from Hell: America in the Age of Genocide*, New York: Basic Books.

Pritchett, Lant (1999) 'Where Has All the Education Gone?' World Bank, Policy Research Working Paper No. 1581.

Quinlan, Tim and Samantha Willan (2005) 'Finding Ways to Contain the HIV/AIDS Epidemic: South Africa 2004–5', in Human Sciences Research Council, *State of the Nation 2004*, Pretoria: HSRC.

Rabwoni, Okwir (2002) 'Reflections on Youth and Militarism in Contemporary Africa', in Alex de Waal and Nicolas Argenti (eds.), *Young Africa: Realising the Rights of Children and Youth*, Trenton NJ: Africa World Press.

Rana, Aziz (2004) 'What Future Democracy?' *Index on Censorship*, 1/04: 56–9.

Reich, Michael (2002) 'Reshaping the State from Above, from Within, from Below: Implications for Public Health', *Social Science and Medicine*, 54: 1669–75.

Richards, Paul (1999) 'Hurry, We Are All Dying of AIDS: Linking Cultural and Agro-technological Responses to the Challenge of Living with AIDS in Africa', unpublished paper, University of Wageningen.

Rosen, Sydney, Ian Sanne, Alizanne Collier and Jonathon L. Simon, (2004) 'Rationing Antiretroviral Therapy for HIV/AIDS in Africa: Efficiency, Equity, and Reality', Boston University Center for International Health and Development, Health and Development Discussion Paper No. 4, February.

Rugalema, Gabriel (2000) 'Coping or Struggling? A Journey into the Impact of HIV/AIDS in Southern Africa', *Review of African Political Economy*, 26: 537–45.

Saunders, Frances Stonor (1999) *Who Paid the Piper? The CIA and the Cultural Cold War*, London: Granta.

Schaffer, Frederic (1998) *Democracy in Translation: Understanding Politics in an Unfamiliar Culture*, Ithaca: Cornell University Press.

Schatzberg, Michael (2001) *Political Legitimacy in Middle Africa: Father, Family, Food*, Bloomington: Indiana University Press, 2001.

Schönteich, Martin (2000) 'Age and AIDS: South Africa's Crime Time Bomb', Pretoria: Institute for Security Studies.

Sen, Amartya K. (1981) *Poverty and Famines: an Essay on Entitlement and Deprivation*, Oxford: Clarendon Press.

—— (1990) 'Individual Freedom as a Social Commitment', *New York Review of Books*, 14 June 1990.

Shilts, Randy (1987) *And the Band Played On: Politics, People and the AIDS Epidemic*, New York: St Martin's Press.

Sontag, Susan (1988) *Illness as Metaphor and AIDS and its Metaphors*, New York: Picador.

Spiegel, Paul (2004) 'HIV/AIDS among Conflict-affected and Displaced Populations', *Disasters*, 28: 322–39.

Ssejoba, Eddie (2004) 'Museveni Condemns Condom Distribution to Pupils', *New Vision* (Kampala), 17 May.

Strand, Per (2005) 'AIDS and Elections in Southern Africa: Is the Epidemic Undermining Its Democratic Remedy?' Institute for Security Studies Paper 110, July.

Strand, Per, Khabele Matlosa, Ann Strode and Kondwani Chirambo (2005) *HIV/AIDS and Democratic Governance in South Africa: Illustrating the Impact on Electoral Processes*, Cape Town: IDASA.

ter Haar, Gerri and Stephen Ellis (2004) *Worlds of Power: Religious Thought and Political Practice in Africa*, London: Hurst.

Tshihamba, Marianne (2001) 'Discrimination of People Living with HIV/

AIDS in Uganda', 3 April, <www.afronets.org/archive/200104/msg 00012.php>, accessed 21 June 2005.

Tumushabe, Joseph (2005) 'The Politics of HIV/AIDS in Uganda', paper for United Nations Research Institute for Social Development, July.

UNAIDS (2004) 'Resource Needs for an Expanded Response to AIDS in Low- and Middle-Income Countries', Geneva: Joint United Nations Programme on HIV/AIDS.

—— (2005) *AIDS in Africa: Three Scenarios to 2025*, Geneva: Joint United Nations Programme on HIV/AIDS.

UNECA (2001) 'Popular Report: African Development Forum 2000: Leadership at All Levels to Overcome HIV/AIDS', Addis Ababa: UN Economic Commission for Africa.

UN IRIN (Integrated Regional Information Networks) (2005) 'Uganda: Back Condom Use, Museveni Urges Catholic Leaders', 15 June.

Urdal, Henrik (2004) 'The Devil in the Demographics: the Effect of Youth Bulges on Domestic Armed Conflict, 1950–2000', World Bank Social Development Papers, Conflict Prevention and Reconstruction, Paper No. 14, July.

Uys, Pieter-Dirk (2004) 'No Laughing Matter', *Index on Censorship*, 1/04: 42–52.

van der Walle, Nicholas (2001) *Africa and the Politics of Permanent Crisis, 1979–1999*, Cambridge: Cambridge University Press.

Vaughan, Megan (1991) *Curing Their Ills: Colonial Power and African Illness*, Stanford: Stanford University Press.

Wallman, Sandra (1996) *Kampala Women Getting By: Wellbeing in the Time of AIDS*, London: James Currey.

Wendo, Charles (2002) 'Uganda Stands Firm on Health Spending Freeze', *The Lancet*, 360 (7 December): 1847.

—— (2003) 'Coverage of HIV/AIDS in the Local News Pages of Ugandan Dailies: a Content Analysis', thesis, Postgraduate Diploma in Mass Communication, University of Makerere, Kampala, Uganda, September.

Whiteside, Alan, Robert Mattes, Samantha Willan and Ryann Manning (2003) 'Examining HIV/AIDS in Southern Africa through the Eyes of Ordinary Southern Africans', Afrobarometer Working Paper No. 21.

Whiteside, Alan, Alex de Waal and Tsadkan Gebre Tensae (2006) 'AIDS, the Military and Security in Africa: a Sober Appraisal', *African Affairs*, forthcoming.

Wiggins, Steve (2005) 'Southern Africa's Food and Humanitarian Crisis of

2001–04: Causes and Lessons', Discussion Paper for Agricultural Economics Society Annual Conference, Nottingham, revised version, 10 May.

Willan, Samantha (2004a) 'Briefing: Recent Changes in the South African Government's HIV/AIDS Policy and Its Implementation', *Journal of African Affairs*, 103: 109–17.

Willan, Samantha (2004b) 'HIV/AIDS, Democracy and Governance in South Africa', GAIN Issue Brief No. 1, <www.justiceafrica.org>.

World Bank (1999) *Confronting AIDS: Public Priorities in a Global Epidemic*, Oxford: Oxford University Press.

Index

Activism 46, 61, 63
AIDS policies 61-2, 64, 95
Policies on Africa 56, 62-3

Wendo, Charles 28-32, 104
Were, Beatrice 51
Willan, Samantha 44, 70
Witchcraft 23-4, 25, 32
World Bank 21, 51, 54, 57, 76,
    79, 86, 103, 104

Youth
    Socialization 83-5
    'Youth bulge' 81

Zambia 13, 15, 25, 55
    Life expectancy 5-6,
    Losses due to AIDS 11
Zimbabwe 18, 20, 55, 121